Frontiers in Anti-Infective Agents
(Volume 4)

(Pregnancy and Anti-Infective Agents)

Edited by

Ricardo Ney Cobucci

Medicine School and Biotechnology Postgraduate Program,
Potiguar University-UnP,
Salgado Filho Av., 1610,
Natal - RN,
Brazil

Frontiers in Anti-Infective Agents

Volume # 4

Pregnancy and Anti-Infective Agents

Editor: Ricardo Ney Cobucci

ISSN (Online): 2705-1080

ISSN (Print): 2705-1072

ISBN (Online): 978-981-14-7959-5

ISBN (Print): 978-981-14-7957-1

ISBN (Paperback): 978-981-14-7958-8

need for a court order if at any point you breach any terms of this License Agreement. In no event will any delay or failure by Bentham Science Publishers in enforcing your compliance with this License Agreement constitute a waiver of any of its rights.

3. You acknowledge that you have read this License Agreement, and agree to be bound by its terms and conditions. To the extent that any other terms and conditions presented on any website of Bentham Science Publishers conflict with, or are inconsistent with, the terms and conditions set out in this License Agreement, you acknowledge that the terms and conditions set out in this License Agreement shall prevail.

Bentham Science Publishers Pte. Ltd.
80 Robinson Road #02-00
Singapore 068898
Singapore
Email: subscriptions@benthamscience.net

BENTHAM SCIENCE

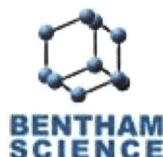

CONTENTS

PREFACE

Bacterial, viral and other infections during pregnancy and breastfeeding not only contribute to maternal morbidity and mortality, but also increase the risk of adverse outcomes including miscarriage, stillbirths, fetal malformation and premature labor.

Currently, the main screened prenatal bacterial and viral infections should be treated with antibiotics and antivirals that contribute to the reduction of adverse outcomes cited.

A concise clinical reference that facilitates the consultation by health professionals regarding the risk classification for use in pregnancy and the puerperium of the main anti-infectious agents indicated in the treatment of prevalent prenatal and postpartum infections was the goal in creating **Pregnancy and anti-infective agents**.

This e-book includes chapters about pharmacodynamics and pharmacokinetics, as well as sexually transmitted and lower genital tract infections in pregnancy and puerperium. It also allows quick consultation on safe antibiotics for the treatment of urinary tract infection and toxoplasmosis in pregnancy. Finally, it innovates in devoting a chapter on promising herbal medicines against infections during pregnancy and breastfeeding.

Ricardo Ney Cobucci
Medicine School and Biotechnology Postgraduate Program,
Potiguar University-UnP,
Salgado Filho Av., 1610,
Natal - RN,
Brazil

List of Contributors

Ada Isa Custódio	Medicine School, Federal University of Rio Grande do Norte, Nilo Peçanha Av., 259 - Petrópolis, Natal RN 59012-310, Brazil
Alexandre Estevam Montenegro Diniz	Medicine School, Potiguar University, Sen. Salgado Filho Av., 1610, Natal, Rio Grande do Norte, Zip Code 59056-600, Brazil
Ana Katherine Gonçalves	Department of Postgraduate Program in Health Sciences, Federal University of Rio Grande do Norte, Natal, Brazil
Ana Paula Costa	Department of Postgraduate Program in Health Sciences, Federal University of Rio Grande do Norte, Natal, Brazil
Antônio Carlos Queiroz de Aquino	Federal University of Rio Grande do Norte, Nilo Peçanha Av., 259, Natal, Brazil
Ayane Cristine Alves Sarmento	Federal University of Rio Grande do Norte, Nilo Peçanha Av., 259, Natal, Brazil
Carolina A. D. Santos	Hospital Giselda Trigueiro, Natal - RN, 59037-170, Brazil Instituto Santos Dumont, Macaíba - RN, 59280-000, Brazil
Diana Gonçalves Dantas	Medicine School and Biotechnology Postgraduate Program, Potiguar University-UnP, 59056-000, Brazil
Fernanda Coêlho Paiva	Medicine School and Biotechnology Postgraduate Program, Potiguar University-UnP, Salgado Filho Av., 1610, Natal - RN, Zip code 59056-000, Brazil
Iaponira da Silva Figueiredo Vidal	Federal University of Rio Grande do Norte, Nilo Peçanha Av., 259, Natal, Brazil
Igor Thiago Queiroz	Hospital Giselda Trigueiro, Natal, Rio Grande do Norte, Brazil
Jaline de Melo Pessoa Cavalcante	Medicine School and Biotechnology Postgraduate Program, Potiguar University-UnP, Salgado Filho Av., 1610, Natal - RN, Zip code 59056-000, Brazil
Janaína Crispim Freitas	Women Health Postgraduate Program and Pharmacy Department, Federal University of Rio Grande do Norte, Natal, Brazil
Juliana Mendonça Freire	Medicine School, Potiguar University, Sen. Salgado Filho Av., 1610, Natal, Rio Grande do Norte, Zip Code 59056-600, Brazil
Júlia Alencar de Medeiros	Medicine School and Biotechnology Postgraduate Program, Potiguar University-UnP, 59056-000, Brazil
Juliana Davim Ferreira Gomes	Medicine School and Biotechnology Postgraduate Program, Potiguar University-UnP, 59056-000, Brazil
Letícia Jales	Medicine School, Federal University of Rio Grande do Norte, Nilo Peçanha Av., 259 - Petrópolis, Natal RN 59012-310, Brazil
Luana Paiva Souza	Medicine School and Biotechnology Postgraduate Program, Potiguar University-UnP, Salgado Filho Av., 1610, Natal - RN, Zip code 59056-000, Brazil
Maria da Conceição Cornetta	Department of Postgraduate Program in Health Sciences, Federal University of Rio Grande do Norte, Natal, Brazil

Matheus de Araújo Duda Medicine School, Potiguar University, Sen. Salgado Filho Av., 1610, Natal, Rio Grande do Norte, Zip Code 59056-600, Brazil

Michelly Nóbrega Monteiro Federal University of Rio Grande do Norte, Nilo Peçanha Av., 259, Natal, Brazil

Mayara Maria Sales Monteiro Medicine School, Federal University of Rio Grande do Norte, Nilo Peçanha Av., 259 - Petrópolis, Natal RN 59012-310, Brazil

Neidmar da Mata Medicine School, Federal University of Rio Grande do Norte, Nilo Peçanha Av., 259 - Petrópolis, Natal RN 59012-310, Brazil

Ricardo Ney Cobucci Medicine School and Biotechnology Postgraduate Program, Potiguar University-UnP, Salgado Filho Av., 1610, Natal - RN, Zip code 59056-000, Brazil

Raniere da Mata Moura Medicine School, Federal University of Rio Grande do Norte, Nilo Peçanha Av., 259 - Petrópolis, Natal RN 59012-310, Brazil

Silvana Maria Zucolotto Medicine School, Federal Univ of Rio Grande do Norte, Natal, Brazil

Themis Rocha Souza Medicine School, Potiguar University, Sen. Salgado Filho Av., 1610, Natal, Rio Grande do Norte, Zip Code 59056-600, Brazil

Wenddy de Lima Cavalcanti Lacerda Medicine School, Federal University of Rio Grande do Norte, Nilo Peçanha Av., 259 - Petrópolis, Natal RN 59012-310, Brazil

CHAPTER 1

Infections in Pregnancy: Maternal and Fetal Risks

Janaína Crispim Freitas, Diana Gonçalves Dantas, Jaline Pessoa Cavalcante, Júlia Alencar de Medeiros, Juliana Davim Ferreira Gomes and **Ricardo Ney Cobucci***

Medicine School and Biotechnology Postgraduate Program, Potiguar University-UnP, Salgado Filho Av., 1610, Natal - RN, Brazil

Abstract: Infections in pregnancy still pose a challenge to public health, especially in less developed countries. They may occur in intrauterine life, and are classified as congenital, or during childbirth and immediate postpartum when they are known as perinatal infections. Infections that occur during pregnancy trigger mechanisms that may culminate in preterm labor, fetal malformations, and fetal and neonatal death. Recognition of signs and symptoms and early diagnosis are the key to reducing the damage that these infections can cause in the mother and the fetus. In this chapter, we will discuss the main infections, risks for maternal and fetal health and strategies that can be used to minimize harm.

Keywords: Cytomegalovirus, Herpes Genitalis, HIV, Infection, Influenza, Parvovirus, Pregnancy, Rubella, Syphilis, Toxoplasmosis.

BACKGROUND

During pregnancy, an immune tolerance is physiologically developed to decrease the chance of fetal rejection. These mechanisms cause increased vulnerability to some infections leading to serious risks for maternal and fetal health [1]. Mother-to-child transmission (MTCT) can occur in intrauterine life, and is classified as congenital, or infections can occur during delivery and immediate postpartum when they are known as perinatal infections [2].

Maternal infections can lead to complications in pregnancy and also in the fetus (Table **1**). Among maternal complications, we have an increased risk of spontan-

---

* **Corresponding author Ricardo Ney Cobucci:** Medicine School and Biotechnology Postgraduate Program, Potiguar University-UnP, Salgado Filho Av., 1610, Natal - RN, Brazil; Tel: +558432151234; E-mail: rncobucci@hotmail.com

eous abortion, premature birth and premature rupture of ovularmembranes. Intrauterine or perinatal infections are a significant cause of fetal and neonatal mortality and contribute to greater early or late childhood morbidity. The infected newborn may exhibit abnormal growth, developmental abnormalities or multiple clinical and laboratory abnormalities [1].

Table 1. Maternal and fetal complications causing by infections in pregnancy.

Maternal Complications	Fetal Complications
• Spontaneous abortion; • Premature birth; • Premature rupture of membranes (PROM); • Secondary infections; • Bacteremia/sepsis;	• Low weight at birth; • Restriction of fetal growth; • Fetal death; • Growth retardation; • Neuro developmental deficits; • Fetal anomalies; • Acute disease after birth; • Asymptomatic infection with late sequelae.

For the most important and common infections, the acronym TORCH is used, which brings together diseases that can have similar clinical manifestations: Toxoplasmosis, Others (syphilis, mumps), Rubella, Cytomegalovirus and Herpes simplex. The concept has recently been expanded to include common pathogens such as enteroviruses, hepatitis viruses, HIV, varicella zoster virus and parvovirus B19 in the "other" category [1, 3].

Several factors, independent of each other, can influence the clinical picture of congenital infections, such as the effect of the pathogen on fetal development, the period of gestational age at which the infection occurred, maternal immunity and the mode of transmission of the infection. Infections that occur in early pregnancy usually cause spontaneous abortions or stillbirths, or may be due to a serious maternal systemic infection [4].

Suspected fetal infection can occur if the mother has been exposed or has an already known infection that can trigger vertical transmission, and it may be possible to detect changes in routine ultrasound exams [4]. In the diagnosis, some tests can be used; one such test is the Polymerase Chain Reaction with Reverse Transcription, which detects the presence of genetic material of the pathogen, and is an exam to be used at the beginning of the infection. After this initial phase of the disease, serological tests become important to assist in the diagnosis. The presence of IgM antibody indicates that there is an active infection, while the IgG antibody indicates a previous contact with the pathogen, which can occur during convalescence or with chronic infection. A method that indicates the time of existence of IgG antibodies is the test of avidity, which in pregnant women has an important role in discovering if the infection occurred before or after conception, and should be performed in the first trimester. A high avidity test means that the infection occurred more than 16 weeks before pregnancy, so there is no need for treatment to prevent fetal transmission [5].

Some clinical cases in the newborn may also suggest an acute congenital infection such as jaundice, petechiae, hepato and/or splenomegaly at birth or immediately after delivery, in a newborn that is unusually small for gestational age (SGA). There may also be the possibility of a congenital infection in the newborn with suspected neonatal sepsis but demonstrating negative cultures for fungi and bacteria [4].

For many of these pathogens, prevention or treatments are available and early recognition, including prenatal screening, is essential. Screening during pregnancy for TOCHA infections varies by location. In the United States, the American College of Obstetricians and Gynecologists (ACOG) recommends screening pregnant women for rubella and syphilis in the first prenatal consultation. In addition to this, some countries also recommend screening for toxoplasmosis during prenatal care [1].

This chapter aims to discuss the main infections acquired during pregnancy, the risks to maternal and fetal health, and the screening, diagnosis and treatment strategies that can be used to minimize the damage.

VIRAL INFECTIONS

Rubella

Rubella is caused by an RNA virus of the *Togavirus* family (*togavirus* and *Rubivirus* genus), with humans acting as its only reservoir. Transmission occurs through direct contact with droplets of nasopharyngeal secretions from an infected individual, its replication occurs in the upper respiratory tract and its dissemination occurs by hematogenous route [6].

Rubella usually has a mild, self-limited and relatively benign clinical picture. However, maternal rubella infection, especially during the first trimester of pregnancy, where there is a high risk of vertical transmission (80-100%), can be catastrophic for the fetus [6]. The infection can result in spontaneous abortion and fetal death or the development of Congenital Rubella Syndrome (CRS) with severe effects on the fetus [3]. The risk decreases in the second quarter (10% - 20%) and increases again close to term (up to 60%) [3].

The MTCT of the rubella virus occurs through hematogenous dissemination during maternal viremia, which usually occurs five to seven days after inoculation of the virus. After infecting the placenta, the virus spreads through the vascular system of the developing fetus and can affect several organs and systems [7].

The classic triad of CRS is characterized by sensorineural deafness, cataracts and cardiac malformations, such as persistence of the artery canal (in 20% of cases) and hypoplasia of the pulmonary artery (12% of cases). These clinical manifestations usually occur if the fetal infection occurs in the first trimester of pregnancy [3].

Cataracts are present in 25% of CRS cases, being bilateral in approximately half of the cases. In addition to cataracts, other ophthalmic abnormalities can occur in around 40% of cases, these include pigmentary retinopathy and glaucoma [8].

The later manifestation of CRS is permanent hearing loss that can appear after two years of life. Hearing loss is usually sensorineural and bilateral and occurs in approximately 80% of patients. It may be the only manifestation of this syndrome, and ranges from mild to severe and may worsen over time [7, 8].

Other cardiovascular disease defects such as pulmonary valve stenosis, aortic valve stenosis, coarctation of the aorta, interatrial communication, interventricular communication and tetralogy of Fallot have also been reported [8].

During the neonatal period, it can cause prematurity, intrauterine growth retardation, microcephaly, radiolucent bone disease, hemolytic anemia, thrombocytopenia, jaundice, hepatitis, hepatomegaly, splenomegaly and purpuric skin lesions. Many of these manifestations are transient and can resolve spontaneously in days or weeks [3].

Rubella is preventable through the measles-mumps-rubella vaccine (MMR); 1 dose of the vaccine is recommended for women of childbearing age who are not immune [3]. CRS is becoming increasingly rare in developed countries with immunization programs against established rubella. However, intermittent rubella outbreaks continue to occur in other parts of the world and CRS remains a concern [6].

With regard to late manifestations, in addition to hearing loss, CRS can also cause psychomotor retardation, speech delay, attention deficit and hyperactivity syndrome, autism, behavioral disorders, progressive encephalopathy, endocrine and immunological disorders [7].

The diagnosis of CRS can be carried out by detecting rubella-specific IgM antibody in serum or umbilical cord blood, which can be more useful until 2 months of age, although in some children, it can be detected until 12 months. The detection of specific IgG in an increasing and persistent form in the serum during the first 7 to 11 months of life can also confirm CRS, but in certain cases, the IgG avidity test can be performed. Rubella virus RNA detected by polymerase chain reaction (PCR) in nasopharyngeal smears, urine, cerebrospinal fluid (CSF) and blood at birth also provides laboratory evidence for the diagnosis of CRS [8].

All newborns with CRS are considered contagious up to at least 1 year of age, unless 2 cultures of clinical samples are negative for rubella virus after 3 months of age [3]. The clinical management of CRS depends on the clinical manifestations that may develop or progress over time, and supportive care and surveillance must be performed. The use of antiviral or biological agents is not recommended, as they do not alter the clinical course of rubella intrauterine infection [9].

Cytomegalovirus

Cytomegalovirus (CMV) is a DNA herpevirus. Cytomegalovirus infection is a common viral infection worldwide and has a stable prevalence of about 4 in 1000 births [10]. The seroprevalence of CMV varies according to population and age. While in developed countries, CMV seroprevalence in women of childbearing age ranges from less than 50 to 85%, in developing countries seroprevalence approaches 100%, this high prevalence can be attributed to exposure through breastfeeding and due to worse conditions of life [11]. Certain factors such as low socioeconomic level, contact with children under 3 years of age, especially if they are in day care, age above 25 to 30 years, greater parity, and living in a developing country increase the prevalence [12].

Transplacental transmission of CMV can occur in women who acquire the first CMV infection in pregnancy (primary infection) or in women with pre-existing antibodies to CMV by reactivating a previous infection or by acquiring a new viral strain [11]. Vertical transmission is higher in pregnant women who have primary infection during pregnancy and the rate of transmission becomes higher with advancing gestational age [12]. In 90% of cases, primary CMV infection during pregnancy is not apparent; however, when it manifests, it shows nonspecific symptoms such as mild fever, rhinitis, pharyngitis, myalgia, arthralgia, headache, and fatigue [12].

Congenital CMV infection is the leading cause of non-hereditary sensorineural hearing loss [1, 13] and it is also associated with long term neurodevelopmental impairment, including cerebral palsy, intellectual disability, visual impairment and seizures [1, 13]. At birth, 85 to 90% of infected babies are asymptomatic and 10 to 15% have a symptomatic disease. In symptomatic children, clinical manifestations include petechiae, jaundice, hepatosplenomegaly, thrombocytopenia, SGA, microcephaly, intracranial calcifications, sensorineural hearing loss, chorioretinitis and seizures [1, 12].

The testing of pregnant women for CMV is indicated when mononucleosis-like diseases are suspected or when a fetal abnormality suggestive of congenital CMV infection is detected in the prenatal ultrasound examination. Seroconversion of IgG specific to CMV is the gold standard for determining primary infections in a previously known non-immune pregnant woman clinically suspected of CMV. However, as pre-conceptual serological screening for CMV is not routinely performed in several countries, seroconversion data is not always available. In the absence of a seroconversion test, IgG avidity detections have been shown to be useful in determining the timing of an infection and, therefore, the risk of intrauterine transmission. Low avidity IgGs are associated with recent infections, between two to four months, while a high avidity index indicates past infections, more than six months ago. However, there are some limitations regarding the use of IgG avidity, as there are still no ideal well established cutoff points for low and high avidity as these vary between laboratories and also commercial avidity antibody assays have variable performance characteristics [14, 15].

Currently, it is recommended to offer invasive (aminocentesis and cordocentesis) and non-invasive (ultrasound and magnetic resonance) methods for prenatal diagnosis when fetal infection is suspected in women with primary infection with high CMV levels [12]. Treatment of symptomatic children with ganciclovir leads to a better prognosis during the first year of life [10].

Herpes Simplex Virus

Herpes simplex virus (HSV) is a DNA virus that is a member of the Herpesviridae family. Neonatal HSV infection occurs in 1 in 3,200 to 10,000 births, and despite the low prevalence of fetal VSH infection it is still worrying, as it can result in great morbidity and mortality [16].

Neonatal HSV has three distinct periods of acquisition: intrauterine, perinatal and postnatal. Intrauterine transmission is very rare. The perinatal represents the majority (85%) of cases and occurs when the pregnant woman has active genital lesions, symptomatic or asymptomatic, during labor. Postnatal represents about 10% of cases and occurs when the newborn maintains contact with oral herpetic lesions of the parent or family member [16].

The manifestations are different according to the area of involvement and can be classified into three main categories. The infection is located only in the eyes, mouth and skin (SEM); it can affect the CNS with or without SEM involvement, or it can occur in a disseminated form in multiple organs [1]. In all categories of neonatal HSV infection, the use of Acyclovir is recommended, being the antiviral agent of choice [17].

Maternal diagnosis is clinical and generally does not require additional tests [18]. In the presence of genital herpes during pregnancy, suppressive antiviral therapy after 36 weeks of gestation may be indicated to reduce the risk of vertical transmission during labor and delivery. However, it is important to mention that no clinical intervention completely eliminates the risk of neonatal herpes infection. The approach with antiviral therapy in pregnant women with HSV is in accordance with ACOG and takes into account the classification of the infection (primary genital herpes, first non-primary genital episode, recurrent herpes), the severity of symptoms, and the time of infection in relation to childbirth [18].

Varicella Zoster Virus

Varicella-zoster virus (VZV) is one of the types of herpesviruses that causes infection in humans. Infection in children is mild and self-limiting, while in adults the disease can progress more severely. In pregnancy, the consequences of chickenpox infection can be a risk for both mother and fetus. It is a very contagious infectious disease transmitted by infected droplets in the nasopharyngeal mucosa or by direct contact with the vesicular secretion containing viruses and, though rare, by the spread of the virus through the air. It may also be transmitted transplacentally causing congenital disease [19].

VZV infection has two clinical manifestations: chickenpox and herpes zoster (HZ). The first is manifested by itchy rashes that start as macules that then develop into papules and then vesicles and can turn into crusted pustules, which can coexist in several different stages of the lesion. After primary infection, VZV is latent in the sensory nerve nodes and can reactivate later in life causing HZ, which is not associated with the occurrence of fetal damage.

In pregnant women, the infection can complicate, leading to meningitis, encephalitis, cerebellar ataxia, pneumonia, secondary bacterial infection, glomerulonephritis, myocarditis, eye disease, adrenal insufficiency and death. Varicella pneumonia is the most common complication in pregnant women and its risk factor is caused by a history of smoking and the presence of more than 100 vesicles on the skin [19].

In the fetus, the early onset of chickenpox at between 8 and 20 weeks has the main consequence of the development of congenital varicella syndrome. Its clinical manifestations are: low birth weight, skin scars that can be depressed and pigmented in a dermatomal distribution; cataract, chorioretinitis, microphthalmia, nystagmus, hypoplastic limbs, cortical atrophy, seizure, gastroesophageal reflux and atretic or stenotic intestine. This syndrome is associated with 30% mortality in the first months of life and a 15% chance of developing HZ by the age of 4 [19].

Maternal diagnosis is clinically based on skin lesions and generally does not require additional tests. Fetal infection can be diagnosed by PCR of fetal blood or amniotic fluid to VZV DNA in conjunction with ultrasound to detect fetal abnormalities. Treatment is carried out with acyclovir. It is important that before conception, women are evaluated if they have immunization for the varicella virus, either by previous infection or immunization by vaccine. In women without previous immunization and who have had contact and been infected with chickenpox, they may receive post-exposure prophylaxis that should be performed with varicella-zoster immunoglobulin [19].

Parvovirus B19

Parvovirus B19 is a single-stranded DNA virus that infects 1 to 5% of pregnant women. It belongs to the *Parvoviridae* family and transmission may occur by respiratory droplets, blood content or transplacental route. The vertical transmission rate is approximately 35% and occurs in 1 to 3 weeks after maternal infection during peak viremia, but the risk of fetal damage is small and of the sequelae is even less [3, 20].

In pregnancy, many women may be asymptomatic. If symptomatic, Parvovirus b19 infection begins with nonspecific symptoms such as fever, malaise, myalgia, and headache. After this stage, there is the appearance of a facial rash known as the chewed face and an itchy macular rash on the trunk, which spreads to the extremities and may be accompanied by polyarthritis. In the fetus, the infection may resolve itself or cause serious damage such as fetal death, severe anemia, non-immune fetal hydrops caused by fetal heart failure, myocardial insufficiency, thrombocytopenia, maternal mirror syndrome and more rarely meningoencephalitis. The risk of an adverse result in the fetus is increased when the infection occurs in the first two months of gestation, the risk is reduced in the second half of pregnancy and is rare in the last 2 months [3, 20].

There is no screening routine for Parvovirus B19, investigation is performed when there are signs of fetal hydrops in the ultrasonography or during the lifetime of symptomatic maternal infection [3]. To confirm the maternal infection, IgM antibody capture radioimmunoassay and enzyme-linked imumunosorbent assay (ELISA) can detect 80-90% of cases with clinical infection, IgM antibody can be detected ten days after the exposure and may persist for three months. To confirm the fetal infection, amniotic or fetal fluid PCR can be used, but viral particles are only detected during the viremia period. In addition, the measurement of IgM antibody in fetal blood can be performed, but the result can be negative even during the surveillance of infection because the fetus only produces IgM after 22 weeks. If fetal death occurs, the diagnosis is made by histopathology [20, 21].

Pregnant women with confirmed infection after 20 weeks of gestation should perform periodic ultrasounds to look for signs of fetal hydrops. However, this procedure is controversial because the risk of fetal harm is low and it is not known whether there is an advantage in monitoring, since the benefit of the intervention is not clear. In fetal management, for a noninvasive investigation of anemia, Doppler assessment of the fetal middle cerebral artery (MCA), peak systolic velocity (PSV) and ductus venosus velocity can be used initially. If severe anemia is detected, cordocentesis should be performed to better assess the anemia and evaluate the indication of intrauterine red blood transfusion. Another approach would be the administration of intravenous immunoglobulin, but there is no formal indication due to limited studies [21].

Influenza

Influenza is a respiratory viral infection caused by the influenza virus, responsible for annual winter epidemics when new strains appear in humans [22]. It is a common and generally self-limiting infection, but complications among pregnant and postpartum women are more prevalent. These occur through cardiopulmonary adaptive changes occurring during pregnancy. These changes include increased heart rate and stroke volume, and reduced pulmonary residual capacity, they may increase the risk of hypoxemia and contribute to the increased severity [23]. There is also an increase in hospitalizations and bed rest in intensive care as well as respiratory diseases mainly in pregnant women with comorbidities such as diabetes, heart problems, chronic renal disease, malignancy and immunosuppression [24, 25]. Historically, the mortality of acute respiratory distress syndrome in pregnancy is high (30% -60%) [26].

The symptoms in pregnant women are similar to those in other populations, and include fever, headache, myalgia, shortness of breath, cough, sore throat and rhinorrhea. The diagnosis is clinical, but some tests can be performed in clinical practice [25]. The test with the greatest specificity and sensitivity is that of RT-PCR, which can differentiate the influenza subtypes. Another alternative is the rapid testing of antigens, but they have a much lower sensitivity [27].

Transplacental transmission of influenza virus is a rare event that appears to be limited to highly pathogenic influenza viruses such as HPAI A and H5N1. However, other serotypes such as H1N1, H2N2 and others have led to increased miscarriages, premature births and maternal mortality during epidemics [24]. Exposure to maternal influenza virus in the first trimester of gestation may be associated with an increased risk of congenital abnormalities such as neural tube defects, hydrocephalus, congenital heart defects, cleft lip, gastrointestinal tract abnormalities and limb defects [16, 25]. The cause of the abnormalities seems to be based on hyperthermia in the embryonic period. However, further research is needed in the area to eliminate confusing elements found in the results [24].

Treatment with antivirals is indicated for pregnant women with suspected or confirmed influenza. Studies have shown that the length of hospital stay was shorter in patients who received therapy in the first 48 hours of symptom onset compared to those who received it after that period. The drugs used in pregnancy are oseltamivir, zanamivir and peramivir for 5 days, but this period may be extended in more severe cases. Oseltamivir is the most used due to its better absorption in the system and to the greater knowledge of its use in pregnant women. Although studies on the safety of these drugs are limited, the benefits of their use outweigh the potential risks. The use of antipyretics is an important possibility since studies have associated fever with fetal damage [25].

The Center for Disease Control (CDC), the Advisory Committee on Immunization Practices (ACIP) and the ACOG recommend that all pregnant women should receive the flu vaccine because of the increased risk of serious illness and complications from infection, furthermore it protects the child in the first months of life [20, 24, 25]. Chemoprophylaxis can be used in pregnant women who have had significant exposure. The main drugs used are zanamivir and oseltamivir for 7 days after the last known exposure [25].

Zika

Zika virus is a flavivurus transmitted mainly by mosquitoes, but it can also be transmitted maternally-fetally, sexually, and through blood transfusion and organ transplants. The RNA of the Zika virus is found in blood, urine, semen, saliva, secretions from the female genital tract, cerebrospinal fluid, amniotic and breast milk, however, this does not define the likelihood of transmission [28]. More recently the zika virus has proved to be dangerous during gestation especially when the infection occurs in the first trimester. Studies in animals and human placentas reinforce the hypothesis that the infection is transmitted by the placenta, moving to the fetal brain and in turn reaching the neuronal progenitor cells and affecting the growth, proliferation, migration and neuronal differentiation. The risk of Zika transmission in pregnancy and estimates of the overall risk of any defect or congenital anomaly between fetuses and babies of women infected with Zika during pregnancy vary widely, probably reflecting differences in the study design [29].

The Royal College of Obstetricians and Gynecologists (RCOG) suggests that the disease consists of two or more symptoms of fever, maculopapular rash, arthralgia and conjunctivitis, however, most people have few symptoms or are asymptomatic. Maternal infection is mild and self-limiting, but it can cause harm to the fetus [30]. Severe congenital anomalies such as microcephaly, facial disproportion, hypertonia/spasticity and hyperflexia, convulsions, irritability, arthrogryposis, ocular abnormalities, sensorineural hearing loss, and neuro-radiological abnormalities (*e.g.*, intracranial calcifications, ventriculomegaly) can be found in the fetuses of infected pregnant women [1]. However, the full spectrum of the syndrome is still being investigated [29].

Diagnostic tests are recommended for pregnant women who have relevant epidemiology and typical symptoms or if an ultrasound exam shows fetal abnormalities compatible with the congenital Zika virus syndrome. In the first 7 days of symptoms the diagnostic test is the RT-PCR for zika virus, after this the serological test (IgM of the zika virus and plaque reduction neutralization test (PRNT)) is indicated. Amniotic fluid RT-PCR can also be performed, but the accuracy of this test is unknown. Another option is that after childbirth a histopathological examination of the placenta and umbilical cord is performed to confirm fetal infection [29].

There is no specific treatment for Zika virus infection, it is consists of controlling maternal symptoms, and there is no therapy to prevent fetal transmission. Prevention is the main way to prevent transmission to the fetus. The pregnant woman must be instructed not to travel to endemic areas, to take protective measures against mosquitos and to use a condom or abstinence to avoid sexual transmission. No vaccine is available yet [29].

Human Immunodeficiency Virus

The global prevalence of Human Immunodeficiency Virus (HIV) makes it one of the most common and deadly diseases worldwide, and of all maternal deaths in the world, 6% to 20% are HIV-related [25]. Many causes of death involve infectious complications from illnesses such as AIDS, tuberculosis, malaria, pneumonia, puerperal sepsis, and sepsis related to spontaneous abortion [26].

In 2013, the US Preventive Services Task Force recommended routine screening of adolescents and adults between 13 to 64 and all pregnant women [26]. The MTCT of human immunodeficiency virus type 1 (HIV-1) can occur in three major periods: *in utero*, at birth, or during breastfeeding. HIV-1 can be transmitted *in utero via* transplacental cellular transport, through a progressive infection of the placenta's trophoblasts until the virus reaches the fetal circulation or due to ruptures in the placental barrier followed by microtransfusions that occur from mother to child. The transmission during delivery occurs *via* the contact of the fetus with infected maternal secretions while passing through the birth canal, through ascending infection from vagina to fetal membranes and amniotic fluid or through absorption in the neonatal digestive tract. In the postpartum period, the main form of transmission is breastfeeding [31].

However, perinatal HIV transmission is almost entirely preventable through a multipronged approach involving universal antenatal HIV screening, careful management of pregnancy including appropriate antiretroviral therapy (ART) and mode of delivery, neonatal antiretroviral prophylaxis, and avoidance of breastfeeding. These interventions have resulted in dramatic reductions in MTCT, and many countries in northern and western Europe have already achieved rates of less than 2%, in line with the WHO goal for virtual elimination of MTCT in the European region by 2015 [32].

The vertical transmission route of HIV-1 can be influenced by several factors, such as the delivery mode, the use of antiretroviral therapy, oral inflammations in the newborn, prematurity, and high maternal viral load. In addition to these factors, the viral genetic diversity appears to play an important role in vertical transmission [31].

Several effects of HIV infection and the combination antiretroviral therapy (cART) on the health of pregnant women and their infants have been described. Since the onset of the HIV epidemic, it has become apparent that maternal HIV infection during pregnancy affects maternal-fetal unity, leading to increased miscarriages, low birth weight, and also increased susceptibility to infections in non-HIV infected infants, who could be exposed. Treatment of pregnant women infected with cART may have a risk of less than or equal to 1-2% MTCT if the maternal viral load is less than or equal to 1000 copies/mL, regardless of the mode of delivery or delivery time or duration of rupture of membranes [20]. Therefore, it is highly recommended that all pregnant women with HIV receive cART with the goal of maximal viral suppression during pregnancy and a consequent decrease in vertical transmission [26].

Pregnant women using cART should have their plasma HIV RNA levels assessed during prenatal care 2 to 4 weeks after starting cART, then monthly until the viral RNA levels are undetectable, and then at least every 3 months during pregnancy [20].

If the viral load is greater than 1000 copies/mL or if the levels are unknown, they should be advised about the benefits of cesarean delivery at 38 weeks of gestational age, in order to reduce the risk of vertical transmission. They should also receive intravenous Zidovudine (ZDV) preoperatively (ideally 3 hours before), followed by continuous infusion for 2 hours until delivery, to achieve adequate levels of the drug in both maternal and fetal blood.

After birth, all newborns of mothers with HIV should receive post-exposure antiviral prophylaxis to decrease the risk of HIV infection, and this should ideally occur within the first 6 to 12 hours after delivery, while the type of prophylaxis will depend on the viremia level of the mother [13].

Rapid screening during labor and delivery or during the immediate postpartum period should be performed for women who have not been tested during pregnancy or whose HIV status is unknown [13].

BACTERIAL INFECTIONS

Syphilis

Syphilis is a sexually transmitted infection (STI) responsible for six million new cases each year in the world, and represents an important public health problem mainly in low and middle income countries. The congenital form occurs by the *Treponema pallidum* passing through the placenta during pregnancy or by contact with an infectious lesion during child-birth. The proportion of congenital cases reflects the number of cases of infection in women of childbearing age [33, 34].

Recognizing the stages of maternal infection is important for early diagnosis and prevention of fetal infection. The first manifestation is the appearance of a painless papule with spontaneous resolution, after 6 to 8 weeks the second stage appears where there is dissemination of eruptions mainly in the palmar and plantar region. The latent stage then occurs, in which women are asymptomatic. If left untreated, maternal syphilis can then progress to the tertiary stage, which is characterized by granulomas affecting the bones and joints as well as the cardiovascular and neurological systems [3]. Risk factors that increase vertical transmission are a lack of adequate prenatal care, high non-treponemal test titers, and late or incomplete treatment [3].

Transplacental transmission can occur at any time during pregnancy, increasing its frequency with increasing gestational age. Pregnant women with untreated primary or secondary syphilis are more prone to vertical transmission than pregnant women with latent disease (60 to 90% *versus* 40% in initial latency and <10% in late latency). The risk of transmission also decreases with the increase in the time of primary or secondary infection, being only 2% after four years of infection. *T. Pallidum* is not transmitted by breast milk, but it is possible if the lactating woman has an infectious lesion in the breast [34].

The manifestations include spontaneous abortion, fetal death, fetal hydrops, and prematurity [1, 3]. However, the majority of newborns may be asymptomatic and come to manifest the clinical picture late in childhood [1]. Symptomatic newborns may have manifestations such as hepatosplenomegaly, nasal secretions, lymphadenopathy, mucosal membrane lesions, pneumonia, osteochondritis, pseudoparalysia, maculopapular eruption, edema, Coombs negative hemolytic anemia and thrombocytopenia [3].

Syphilis of the central nervous system (CNS) in children with congenital infection is most often asymptomatic, and is indicated by abnormalities in the cerebrospinal fluid. Symptomatic involvement is rare, and can only be found in children not treated in the neonatal period. There are two types of presentation: acute syphilitic leptomeningitis and chronic meningovascular syphilis. The first one is manifested in the first year of life, mainly between three and six months, and the clinical findings are suggestive of bacterial meningitis infection, although with findings of aseptic meningitis in the cerebrospinal fluid. Chronic meningovascular syphilis manifests at the end of the first year of life with clinical findings including progressive hydrocephalus, cranial nerve palsies, papilledema, optic atrophy, neurodevelopmental regression, and seizures [33].

The Venereal Disease Research Laboratory test (VDRL) or the rapid plasma reagin test are used for screening during prenatal care and appropriate treatment is given with intramuscular (IM) penicillin during pregnancy, patients allergic to penicillin should be desensitized [3]. Screening and treatment of syphilis are recognized as one of the most economical public health interventions available and can prevent the onset of congenital syphilis [34].

Group B Streptococcus

Group B streptococcus (GBS) is an encapsulated gram-positive coccus that often causes risks to maternal and fetal health. It colonizes human genital and gastrointestinal tracts and the upper respiratory tract of young infants. Transmission occurs upwardly from the vagina to the amniotic fluid. It can occur either at the onset of labor with the rupture of membranes or during the passage through the birth canal [35].

Damage caused by GBS in pregnant women includes urinary tract infection, upper genital tract infection, intra-amniotic infection, endometritis and bacteremia. Invasive maternal infection is associated with miscarriage and preterm labor [36]. The importance of screening and prophylaxis is due to the damage it can cause in the newborn. GBS remains the leading cause of neonatal sepsis and meningitis in human newborns during the first week of life [35].

The ACOG in 2019 recommended that rectovaginal screening cultures for GBS be performed on all pregnant women from 36 weeks to 37 weeks and 6 days, with the exception of women with GBS bacteriuria during their current pregnancy or who have undergone previous pregnancies with the child infected with GBS, because these have already had the indication for prophylactic treatment [36].

Intrapartum antibiotic prophylaxis is indicated for all patients who have a positive screening culture for GBS in the vagina or rectum, history of previous pregnancy with GBS infection of the newborn, bacteriuria by GBS during current pregnancy or that the culture for GBS is unknown and associated with intrapartum fever, premature labor, preterm rupture of membranes or prolonged rupture of membranes ≥18 hours. Prophylaxis must be performed intravenously so that the antibiotic reaches the fetal circulation and must be started at least four hours before delivery. The most used antibiotics are penicillin G or ampicillin is indicated in cases of mild allergy to cefazolin and in cases of severe allergies clindamycin or erythromycin is used. Prophylaxis is not indicated for patients undergoing cesarean section [37]. There are still no licensed vaccines, however, the results of vaccine clinical trials are promising [36].

OTHER INFECTIONS

Toxoplasmosis

Toxoplasmosis is a disease caused by infection of the protozoan *Toxoplasma gondii* (*T. gondii*). It is transmitted through the ingestion of parasitic cysts that are in the environment, found in raw or undercooked meat or by transfusion of blood products and organ transplantation [3, 17]. There are three genotypes (I, II, III) of *T. gondii*. Type II is the predominant strain responsible for up to 80% of congenital infections in Europe and the United States [3].

Congenital infection occurs through the transplacental transmission of *T. gondii* after maternal primary infection when there is high parasitemia [3]. Non-immune pregnant women have a variable risk of between 10 and 100% transmission [10].

The risk of transmission is higher at the end of gestation, however, during this time the clinical manifestations in the baby are less severe [10, 17]. Although rare, infection in early pregnancy can lead to severe complications [10, 17].

In most cases, congenital toxoplasmosis is asymptomatic, but in some cases, it manifests itself with the classic triad consisting of chorioretinitis, hydrocephalus and intracranial calcifications. Other signs such as fever, maculopapular rash, hepatosplenomegaly, microcephaly, convulsions, jaundice, thrombocytopenia and generalized lymphadenopathy accompany the disease [1]. Chorioretinitis, microcephaly, seizures, intellectual disability and sensorineural hearing loss may manifest only as late sequelae in newborns born with no signs and symptoms [3].

There is no universal standard for screening pregnant women for toxoplasmosis. The most used tests for diagnosis in pregnant women are serological IgM (there is a high rate of false positives) and IgG. The RT-PCR of maternal blood is seldom used. The avidity test should be performed for patients with positive IgM and IgG, to investigate whether maternal infection occurred before or after conception. A high avidity test does not require treatment to prevent fetal transmission [5]. A positive result of amniotic fluid by PCR before 18 weeks can determine fetal infection [3].

Treatment initiated up to 18 weeks after gestation begins with spiramycin, and if PCR and ultrasound results are available and fetal infection is confirmed, treatment changes to sulfadiazine, pyrimethamine, folinic acid, and spiramycin [3].

The postnatal investigation is done with IgG, IgM and IgA, CSF if indicated and PCR in addition to ophthalmological, auditory and neurological examinations. Computed tomography of the head is the preferred method of visualizing intracranial calcifications. Postnatal treatment consists of 12 months of pyrimethamine, sulfadiazine and folinic acid to minimize hematologic toxicity associated with pyrimethamine. It is recommended that the test is repeated 1 month after discontinuation of therapy. Close and sequential follow-up with serial eye exams, as well as auditory and neurological exams, is the key to recognizing sequelae of this disease [3].

CONCLUSION

Infections during pregnancy have been associated with adverse pregnancy outcomes and birth defects in the offspring. Those acquired by the fetus in the womb or during the labor process are a significant cause of fetal and neonatal mortality and an important contributor to early and late childhood morbidity.

Many of the agents have specific screening available to perform during prenatal care, early recognition allows for proper treatment, minimizing maternal and fetal damage. Vaccination is an effective and cost-effective tool to reduce preventable congenital infectious diseases.

Pregnant women and their infants present vulnerabilities that should receive constant vigilance. Pre-natal follow-up is essential to reduce adverse outcomes. Physicians who follow up should always be aware of the most common presentations, appropriate diagnostic approaches, and available therapies.

CONSENT FOR PUBLICATION

Not applicable.

CONFLICT OF INTEREST

The authors declare no conflict of interest, financial or otherwise.

ACKNOWLEDGEMENTS

Declared None.

REFERENCES

[1]   Johnson KEJ. Overview of TORCH infections. In: Weisman LE, Edwards MS, Armsby C, Eds. [revised Sep 2020; cited 20st Dec 2018] 2019. Available from: https://www.uptodate.com/ contents/overview-of-torch-infections

[2]   Madrid L, Varo R, Sitoe A, Bassat Q. Congenital and perinatally-acquired infections in resource-constrained settings. Exp Rev Anti-infect Ther 2016; 14(9): 845-61. Available from: https://www.tandfonline.com/doi/full/10.1080/14787210.2016. 1215913 [http://dx.doi.org/10.1080/14787210.2016.1215913] [PMID: 27442227]

[3]   Neu N, Duchon J, Zachariah P. TORCH infections. Clinics in Perinatology 2015; 42(1): 77-103. Available from: https://www.sciencedirect.com/science/article/abs/pii/S0095510814001250?via%3Di hub [http://dx.doi.org/10.1016/j.clp.2014.11.001] [PMID: 25677998]

[4]   Cofre F, Delpiano L, Labraña Y, Reyes A, Sandoval A, Izquierdo G. TORCH syndrome: Rational approach of pre and post natal diagnosis and treatment. Recommendations of the Advisory Committee on Neonatal Infections Sociedad Chilena de Infectología. Rev Chil Infectol 2016; 33(2): 191-216. Available from: https://scielo.conicyt.cl/scielo.php?script=sci_arttext&pid=S0716-101820160002000 10&lng=en. [http://dx.doi.org/10.4067/S0716-10182016000200010]

[5]   Schwartzman JD, Petersen E. Diagnostic testing for toxoplasmosis infection. In: Weller PF, Mitty J, Eds. [revised Sep 2020; cited 26st Jul 2020] 2019. Available from: https://www.uptodate.com/ contents/diagnostic-testing-for-toxoplasmosis-infection

[6]   Riley L. Rubella in pregnancy. In: Hirsch MS, Lockwood CJ, Bloom A, Eds. 2019. Available from: https://www.uptodate.com/contents/rubella-in-pregnancy

[7]   Leung AKC, Hon KL, Leong KF. Rubella (German measles) revisited. Hong Kong Med J 2019; 25(2): 134-41. Available from: https://www.hkmj.org/abstracts/v25n2/134.htm

[8]   Dobson S. Congenital rubella syndrome: clinical features and diagnosis. In: Edwards MS, Weisman LE, Armsby C, Eds. 2018. Available from: https://www.uptodate.com/contents/congenital-rubell--syndromeclinical- features-and-diagnosis

[9]   Dobson S. Congenital rubella syndrome: Management, outcome, and prevention. In: Edwards MS, Weisman LE, Armsby C, Eds. 2020. Available from: https://www.uptodate.com/contents/congenital-rubella-syndromemanagement-outcome-and-p revention

[10]   Ville Y, Leruez-Ville M. Managing infections in pregnancy. Curr Opin Infect Dis 2014; 27(3): 251-7. Available from: https://journals.lww.com/co-infectiousdiseases/Abstract/2014/06000/Managing_infections_in_pregnancy.7.aspx
[http://dx.doi.org/10.1097/QCO.0000000000000066] [PMID: 24781057]

[11]   Marsico C, Kimberlin DW. Congenital Cytomegalovirus infection: advances and challenges in diagnosis, prevention and treatment. Ital J Pediatr 2017; 43(38) Available from: https://www.ncbi.nlm.nih.gov/pmc/articles/PMC5393008/
[http://dx.doi.org/10.1186/s13052-017-0358-8] [PMID: 28416012]

[12]   Sheffield JS, Boppana SB. Cytomegalovirus infection in pregnancy. In: Wilkins-Haug K, Hirsch MS, Barss VA, Eds. 2020. Available from: https://www.uptodate.com/contents/cytomegalovirus-infection-in-pregnancy

[13]   Hughes B, Cu-Uvin S. Intra-labor management of pregnant women with HIV and child prophylaxis in resource-rich environments. In: Mofenson, LM, Bloom A, Eds. 2020. Available from: https://www.uptodate.com/contents/intrapartum-management-of-pregnant-women-with-hiv-and-infant-prophylaxis-in-resource-rich-settings

[14]   Sheffield JS, Boppana SB. Cytomegalovirus infection in pregnancy. In: Wilkins-Haug L, Hirsch MS, Barss VA, Eds. 2020. Available from: https://www.uptodate.com/contents/cytomegalovirus-infection-in-pregnancy

[15]   Saldan A, Forner G, Mengoli C, Gussetti N, Palù G, Abate D. Testing for Cytomegalovirus in Pregnancy. J Clin Microbiol 2017; 55(3): 693-702. Available from: https://www.ncbi.nlm.nih.gov/pmc/articles/PMC5328437/
[http://dx.doi.org/10.1128/JCM.01868-16] [PMID: 28031434]

[16]   Demmeler-Harrison GJ. Neonatal herpes simplex virus infection: Clinical features and diagnosis. In: Sheldon L Kaplan, Leonard E Weisman, Eds. 2018. Available from: https://www.uptodate.com/contents/neonatal-herpes-simplex-virus-infection-clinical-features-and-diagnosis

[17]   Demmeler-Harrison GJ. Neonatal herpes simplex virus infection: Management and prevention. In: Sheldon L Kaplan, Leonard E Weisman, Eds. 2018. Available from: https://www.uptodate.com/contents/neonatal-herpes-simplex-virus-infection-management-and-prevention

[18]   Riley LE. Varicella-zoster virus infection in pregnancy. In: Martin S Hirsch, Charles J Lockwood, Eds. 2019. Available from: https://www.uptodate.com/contents/varicella-zoster-virus-infection-in-pregnancy

[19]   Riley L, Wald A. Infecção pelo vírus herpes simplex genital e gravidez. In: Martin S Hirsch, Charles J Lockwood, Eds. 2020. Available from: https://www.uptodate.com/contents/neonatal-herpes-simpl-x-virusinfection-clinical-features-and-diagnosis

[20]   Labor and Delivery Management of Women With Human Immunodeficiency Virus Infection. American College of Obstetricians and Gynecologists (ACOG) 2018; 132(3): e131-7. Available from: https://www.acog.org/-/media/project/acog/acogorg/clinical/files/committee-opinion/articles/2018/09/labor-and-delivery-management-of- women-with-hiv-infection.pdf

[21]   Riley L, Fernandes C. Parvovirus B19 infection during pregnancy. In: Martin S Hirsch, Morven S Edwards, Leonard E Weisman, Eds. 2020. Available from: https://www.uptodate.com/contents/parvovirus-b19-infection-during-pregnancy

[22]   Gabas T, Leruez-Ville M, Le Mercier D, Lortholary O, Lecuit M, Charlier C. Grippe et grossesse

[Influenza and pregnancy]. Presse Med 2015; 44(6 Pt 1): 639-46. Available from: https://www.researchgate.net/publication/277337824_ Grippe_et_grossesse [http://dx.doi.org/10.1016/j.lpm.2015.04.012] [PMID: 26033556]

[23]   Kourtis AP, Read JS, Jamieson DJ. Pregnancy and infection. N Engl J Med 2014; 370(23): 2211-8. Available from: https://www.nejm.org/doi/full/10.1056/nejmra1213566 [http://dx.doi.org/10.1056/NEJMra1213566] [PMID: 24897084]

[24]   Ghulmiyyah LM, Alame MM, Mirza FG, Zaraket H, Nassar AH. Influenza and its treatment during pregnancy: A review. J Neonatal Perinatal Med 2015; 8(4): 297-306. Available from: https://pubmed.ncbi.nlm.nih.gov/26012384/ [http://dx.doi.org/10.3233/NPM-15814124] [PMID: 26836818]

[25]   Jamieson D J, Rasmussen S A. Seasonal influenza and pregnancy. In: Vincenzo Berghella, Martin S Hirsch, Eds. 2020. Available from: https://www.uptodate.com/contents/seasonal-influenza -andpregnancy

[26]   Eppes C. Management of Infection for the Obstetrician/Gynecologist. Obstet Gynecol Clin North Am 2016; 43(4): 639-57. Available from: https://pubmed.ncbi.nlm.nih.gov/ 27816152/ [http://dx.doi.org/10.1016/j.ogc.2016.07.009] [PMID: 27816152]

[27]   Dolin R. Diagnosis of seasonal influenza in adults. 2019. Available from: https://www.uptodate.com/ contents/diagnosis-of- seasonal-influenza-in-adults

[28]   LaBeaud AD. Zika virus infection: An overview. In: Martin S Hirsch, Ed. 2020. Available from: https://www.uptodate.com/contents/zika-virus-infe ction-an-overview

[29]   Lockwood CJ, Ros ST, Nielsen-Saines K. Zika Virus Infection: Evaluation and Management of Pregnant Women. In: Hirsch MS, Levine D, Simpson LL, Eds. . Available from: https://www.uptodate.com/contents/zika-virus-infection-evaluation-and-managementof-pregnant-women

[30]   Lissauer D, Smit E, Kilby MD. Zika virus and pregnancy. BJOG 2016; 123(8): 1258-63. Available from: https://obgyn.onlinelibrary.wiley.com/full/10. 1111doi//1471-0528.14071 [http://dx.doi.org/10.1111/1471-0528.14071] [PMID: 27150456]

[31]   Rosa MC, Lobato RC, Gonçalves CV, *et al.* Evaluation of factors associated with vertical HIV-1 transmission. J Pediatr (Rio J) 2015; 91(6): 523-8. Available from: https://pubmed.ncbi.nlm. nih.gov/26126701/ [http://dx.doi.org/10.1016/j.jped.2014.12.005] [PMID: 26126701]

[32]   Townsend CL, Byrne L, Cortina-Borja M, *et al.* Earlier initiation of ART and further decline in mother-to-child HIV transmission rates, 2000-2011. AIDS 2014; 28(7): 1049-57. Available from: https://pubmed.ncbi.nlm.nih.gov/24566097/ [http://dx.doi.org/10.1097/QAD.0000000000000212] [PMID: 24566097]

[33]   Dobson S. Congenital syphilis: clinical features and diagnosis. In: L Kaplan, Leonard E Weisman, Eds. 2019. Available from: https://www.uptodate.com/contents/congenital-syphilis-clinicalfeatur-s-and-diagnosis

[34]   Trinh TT, Kamb ML, Luu M, Ham DC, Perez F. Syphilis testing practices in the Americas. Trop Med Int Health 2017; 22(9): 1196-203. Available from: https://pubmed.ncbi.nlm.nih.gov/28653418/ [http://dx.doi.org/10.1111/tmi.12920]

[35]   Melin P. Neonatal group B streptococcal disease: from pathogenesis to preventive strategies. Clin Microbiol Infect 2011; 17(9): 1294-303. Available from: https://pubmed.ncbi.nlm.nih.gov/21672083/ [http://dx.doi.org/10.1111/j.1469-0691.2011.03576.x] [PMID: 21672083]

[36]   Puopolo KM, Madoff LC, Baker CJ. Group B Streptococcal Infection in Pregnant Women. In: Daniel J Sexton, Ed. . Available from: https://www.uptodate.com/contents/group-b-streptococcalinfection-in-pregnant-women

[37]   Karen MP, Baker CJ. Neonatal Group B Streptococcal Disease. In: Edwards MS, Ed. 2019. Available from: https://www.uptodate.com/contents/neonatal-group-b-streptococcal-disease-pre- vention

Pharmacodynamics and Pharmacokinetics of Anti-Infective Agents in Pregnant Women

Neidmar da Mata[1,*], Letícia Jales[1], Ada Isa Custódio[1], Mayara Maria Sales Monteiro[2], Wenddy de Lima Cavalcanti Lacerda[2] and Raniere da Mata Moura[1]

[1] *Medicine School, Federal University of Rio Grande do Norte, Nilo Peçanha Av., 259 Petrópolis, Natal-RN, 59012-310, Brazil*

[2] *Medicine School, Potiguar University, Natal-RN, Brazil*

Abstract: Pregnancy is considered a special moment in a woman's life. However, in this period, physiological changes take place that make the woman more vulnerable to infectious agents. The use of medications in this period may pose risks to both the mother and the developing infant, and subsequently, common physiological changes interfere greatly with the dynamics and kinetics of the drugs. There is still a concern about possible toxic effects on the mother and fetus as well as possible teratogeny. This chapter aims to discuss the anti-infective agents to broaden the understanding of the fundamental concepts, practical applications of the drugs prescribed and the necessary care for pregnant women.

Keywords: Anti-infective agents, Antifungal, Antibiotics, Antiviral, Birth outcomes, Congenital defects, Pharmacology, Pregnant women, Teratogenicity, Therapy.

BACKGROUND

Infections in pregnancy are the third most common cause of maternal mortality, accounting for approximately 10% of maternal deaths [1, 2]. Sepsis is the main cause of deaths related to infection, and its prevention, early diagnosis and appropriate management are essential to reduce maternal morbidity and mortality [1].

Multiple biological, cultural, and social factors are responsible for the increased susceptibility to infection and the subsequent poorv outcomes. These factors also

* **Corresponding address Neidmar da Mata**: Medicine School, Federal University of Rio Grande do Norte, Nilo Peçanha Av., 259 - Petrópolis, Natal - RN, 59012-310, Brazil; Tel: +5584 3215 1234; E-mail: neidmar@gmail.com

Ricardo Ney Cobucci (Ed.)

alter the presentation of infectious syndromes and may require changes in treatment [3].

Infections in the pregnant woman represent a risk to the mother's health and the development of the fetus. They can lead to premature rupture of membranes and thus increase the risk of miscarriage and prematurity. Also, certain infectious agents can cross the placental barrier and directly affect the fetus. Therefore, an anti-infective treatment should be effective and safe for both mother and fetus [4, 5].

Pregnancy is a special condition, with many physiological changes taking place that may influence drug behavior, and which may have an impact on the disposition and effectiveness of drugs.

Anti-infective agents are among the most commonly prescribed medications for pregnant women. However, the use of these drugs poses several challenges in this population. There is a lack of research, especially clinical trials, dedicated to this group of patients [6]. There is also the need to consider the adverse risk effects of drugs on pregnancy and fetal development (allergic reactions, disorders in various systems, teratogenicity and death) [7]. In addition, the long-term implications of side effects should be considered when exposure to the drug occurs in the early stages of life.

There are significant differences in the pharmacokinetics of anti-infective agents due to the physiological adaptations that occur during pregnancy which complicate the selection of an optimal dosage regimen [6]. These physiological differences coupled with the scarcity of pharmacokinetic data, result in considerable uncertainty about treatment recommendations. The efficacy of many anti-infective agents is determined by an exposure-response relationship (Fig. **1**) [6, 8].

These drugs may exhibit a dependency (Cpmax/minimum inhibitory concentration (MIC)), have a time-dependent (T> MIC) concentration and/or be exposure dependent on the death of microorganisms (Area under the curve (AUC)/MIC) [6].

To reach the systemic circulation, the drug must cross membranes and overcome the enzymatic repertoire that can inactivate it in different compartments. The term bioavailability is used to denote the fraction of an oral dose that reaches the systemic circulation in the form of an intact drug, taking into account both absorption and local metabolic degradation [9]. Bioavailability is not a characteristic of drugs alone, variations in pH and enzymatic activities in the gastric, intestinal or hepatic systems should also be considered. Physiological changes in pregnancy influence the behavior of most drugs [10, 11]. An understanding of these natural changes may help the practitioner anticipate changes in the pharmacological behavior of a drug, consequently modifying its dosage to achieve the desired pharmacodynamic effects. Studies have shown that pregnant women use an average of 2 to 5 medications throughout pregnancy [10, 12]. The most common agents used by women in the first trimester of pregnancy are antibiotics and vaccines [13, 14].

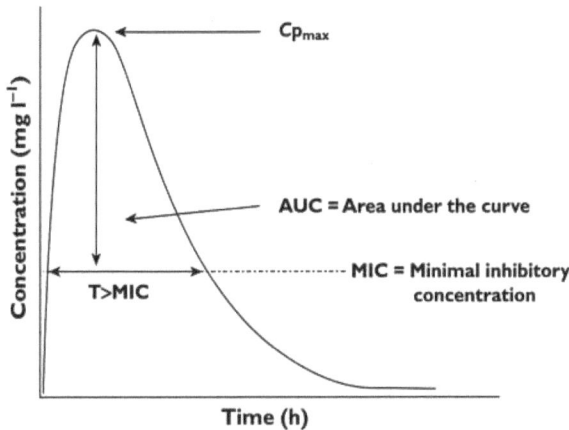

Fig. (1). Pharmacokinetic parameters affecting organism killing.

Here, we specifically focus on anti-infective agents for seeking an understanding of the concepts, their practical applications and care in pregnant women.

PHARMACOLOGICAL CONSIDERATIONS AND PHYSIOLOGICAL CHANGES DURING PREGNANCY

Pharmacokinetics and Pharmacodynamics

Pharmacodynamic aspects are determined by processes such as drug-receptor interaction which are specific for the drug class [9]. In turn, pharmacokinetics refers to the movement of the drug in the body, describing its absorption, distribution, metabolism and elimination, *i.e.*, what the body does with the drug [15]. The concept of these processes is summarized in Table **1**. The type of response of an individual to a particular drug depends on the pharmacological properties inherent to the drug at its site of action. However, the speed of onset, intensity and duration of response generally depend on parameters such as [9]:

a. the rate and extent of absorption of the drug from its site of administration;
b. the rate and extent of drug distribution to different tissues including the site of action;
c. the rate of elimination of the drug from the body.

Each part of this pathway can be affected by numerous physiological changes, which in turn, significantly affect dosage regimens [10].

Table 1. Principles of Pharmacokinetics [15].

Absorption	Movement of the medicine from its place of administration into the bloodstream. It depends on physico-chemical properties, formulation and route of administration of the drug
Distribution	Delivery of the drug to body tissues. Variables such as tissue blood flow, capillary permeability and tissue volume affect the rate of distribution and amount of drug in tissue
Metabolism	Process of transformation of drugs in order to facilitate their elimination from the body. This occurs mainly in the liver and involves phase 1 (oxidation, reduction or hydrolysis) and phase 2 (conjugation with a second molecule) reactions
Excretion	Elimination of the drug from the body, either unchanged or as a metabolite. The kidney is the most important organ in this phase

Drug Absorption

The physical processes of diffusion, passing through membranes, binding to plasma proteins and partition between adipose tissue and other tissues are the basis of drug absorption and distribution.

Absorption of the drug in the circulatory system depends on the route of administration (oral, subcutaneous, intramuscular, intravenous, inhalation, transdermal, vaginal or rectal). The altered behavior of the drug due to changes in maternal physiology may influence the bioavailability of the drug and the proportion of drug administered that reaches the systemic circulation in intact form [10]. Although it is a parameter related to absorption, it does not apply to an intravascularly administered drug. Therefore, by definition, an intravenously administered drug is 100% bioavailable. That is, the entire dose of the drug is administered directly into the circulatory chain and is available to interact with the receptors and trigger the pharmacological effect. The oral route (VO) of drug administration is one of the most commonly employed during pregnancy. The effects of medications taken orally may be affected by several factors, including stomach pH, food, intestinal transit time, local intestinal metabolism, intestinal microbiota, transport of uptake and efflux transport, and pre-systemic metabolism. In the general population, the amount of intact drug that reaches the systemic circulation after being metabolized is greatly reduced. In the pregnant woman, there is an elevation of the gastric pH, which can cause greater ionization of weak acids and compromise the absorption. In addition, endogenous progesterone decreases intestinal mobility, increasing orocecal transit time and increasing absorption [10, 16]. Throughout the third trimester of pregnancy, blood volume increases from 40% to 45% above the non-gravid state, resulting in a greater volume of distribution of hydrophilic drugs such as piperacillin, metformin and tenofovir. This volumetric growth also translates into a pre-systemic effect, reducing bioavailability. A higher rate of glomerular filtration (GFR) can also be observed, resulting in a greater renal clearance of drugs such as atenolol, digoxin, metformin and cefuroxime. There is also the secondary effect of reducing albumin and acid α1-glycoproteins, leading to a higher proportion of free fraction with critical repercussions for drugs with high affinity for plasma proteins such as phenytoin and tracolimus [10, 17].

Thus, due to the many variables that affect the absorption of oral medications, there is a wide variation in plasma levels leading to clinical variations and possible undesirable effects [10].

During pregnancy, sexually transmitted infections or untreated urinary tract infections are associated with significant morbidity, including low birth weight, preterm birth, and miscarriage [5]. About one in four women is prescribed an antibiotic during pregnancy which accounts for almost 80% of the drugs prescribed for pregnant women [5]. Exposure to antibiotics during pregnancy has been linked in the short term to congenital and long-term anomalies such as changes in the intestinal microbiome, asthma and atopic dermatitis in the newborn. However, it is estimated that only 10% of medicines have enough data related to safe and effective use in pregnancy. Beta-lactam antibiotics such as vancomycin, nitrofurantoin, clindamycin, fosfomycin and metronidazole are generally considered safe and effective in pregnancy. On the other hand, fluoroquinolones and tetracyclines are generally avoided in pregnancy [18].

Drug Distribution

The distribution is the transfer of the medicine from the general circulation to the different organs of the body [9]. The volume of distribution (Vd = total drug in the body/drug in plasma) is the theoretical volume occupied by the drug if it dissolves homogeneously throughout the body and its concentration in all parts is equal to that of plasma. The Vd estimates the total amount of drug in the body, *i.e.,* the extravascular extent in the dynamic equilibrium phase. If a drug is highly bound to the tissue, the Vd will be very large. A large Vd means a lower plasma concentration by the localization of the drug in the receptors of the tissues (extravascular space). When there is a great loss of blood volume, drugs with a large Vd are more likely to remain in the body (greater extravascular distribution) as compared to the drugs with a small Vd (mainly intravascular). An additional unique feature of pregnancy is the transplacental transfer of medications to the fetal compartment (fetus, amniotic fluid, gestational tissues). The passage of a drug into the fetal compartment is reflected by a higher Vd than that in the non-gestational state, mainly due to the distribution in the amniotic fluid [10]. An increase in Vd may modify the efficacy of anti-infectives by decreasing the drug at maternal receptor sites while increasing fetal exposure. The distribution of a drug depends on several factors which include tissue perfusion level, plasma protein binding, liposolubility, vascular permeability, tissue binding, and organic barriers. Many of these factors are altered in pregnancy, usually leading to increased drug distribution. In addition, pregnancy is a state of hypoalbuminemia, as previously reported, which provides a greater free fraction of the drug, decreasing it at the receptor site. Significant hemodynamic changes during pregnancy occur due to increased activity of the renin-angiotensin-aldosterone system, resulting in greater retention of Na^{++} and H_2O. This contributes to increased blood flow and tissue perfusion, increasing cardiac output by 30% to 50%, which in turn increases the volume and heart rate, altering the regional blood flow and favoring the perfusion of the pelvic organs. Blood flow to the uterus, kidneys, skin and mammary glands increases during pregnancy while blood flow to the muscles decreases, resulting in increased Vd for most drugs with a preferential exposure of the drug to the reproductive organs [10].

As most drugs cross the placenta, care must be taken in their use during pregnancy because of the possibility of causing teratogenesis or other damage to the fetus. Despite this known risk, there are few studies with scientific evidence on the use of drugs during pregnancy due to the involved ethical issues. Therefore, current knowledge about the safety of known drugs stems from studies in which pregnant women were not excluded from new therapies or from data extracted from animal models and observational studies [19, 20]. Lipophilic drugs are known to cross the placental barrier rapidly as compared to hydrophilic agents which limits exposure of the fetus to the drug after a single maternal dose. Hydrophilic agents such as low molecular weight heparins can be effectively excluded by the placental barrier without causing any effects to the fetus, if administered chronically to the mother.

Drug Metabolism

The metabolism of a drug describes the range of biochemical modifications performed by specialized enzyme systems to facilitate excretion [10]. Drug metabolism involves two types of reactions, known as phase 1 and phase 2, and they often occur sequentially. Both phases decrease liposolubility, thus increasing renal elimination. Phase 1 reactions (*e.g.*, oxidation, reduction or hydrolysis) are catabolic and their products are generally chemically more reactive; therefore, paradoxically, they sometimes become more toxic or carcinogenic than the original drug. The liver is especially important at this stage, in which metabolic actions involve enzymes of the cytochrome P450 family (CYP), and flavin monooxygenases. Activation of metabolic enzymes is highly variable and is affected by a number of factors, such as race, ethnicity, age, concomitant medications and pregnancy. High hepatic blood flow in pregnancy increases drug exposure to enzyme metabolism, promoting pre-systemic metabolism, requiring a much higher dose of the drug when given orally than parenterally. Changes in the hormonal environment in pregnancy, increase the activity of some enzymes, such as CYP34A, -2C9, -2D9 and decrease the activity of others, such as CYP1A2 [10]. It should also be remembered that the efficacy of the drug-metabolizing enzymes in the liver of the adult woman is greater than in the liver of the fetus. A detailed understanding of the enzymatic metabolism of a given drug during pregnancy is crucial to predict adjustments in drug concentrations to achieve pharmacodynamic targets [10]. Phase 2 reactions are synthetic (anabolic) and include conjugation (*i.e.,* binding of a substituent group), which normally results in inactive products, although there are exceptions. Phase 2 reactions occur primarily in the liver. If the drug molecule or a phase 1 product has a suitable radical (*e.g.*, a hydroxyl, thiol or amino group), it becomes susceptible to conjugation. The chemical group is inserted may be glucuronyl, sulfate, methyl or acetyl. Glutathione, as another example, conjugates drugs or their phase 1 metabolites through the hydrogen sulfide group [21].

Elimination of Drugs

Elimination is the final step of drug distribution in the body. It consists of the process by which a drug is excreted unchanged or after modification by metabolites. Common elimination routes are the kidneys, liver, skin, lungs, feces, and glands (mammary, lacrimal, salivary, sweat). Changes in the elimination of a drug result in the accumulation of the original drug or its metabolites. In pregnancy, the above-mentioned cardiovascular changes including increased cardiac output (increased systolic and heart rate) and preferential regional blood flow, contribute to increased clearance of the drug. Increased hepatic and renal blood flow due to decreased renal vascular resistance also contribute to increased elimination. Renal elimination is the main route of drug elimination, although elimination can also be done through the lungs as well. Pregnant women have increased breathing and decreased functional reserve capacity which leads to reduced PCO_2 and therefore, compensatory respiratory alkalosis. These factors contribute to increased lung clearance of inhaled drugs. Another important factor in elimination is the concomitant use of drugs whose drug interactions or metabolic induction/enzymatic inhibition may affect the rate of elimination of the drug involved [10]. It is noteworthy that the fetal kidney is not an efficient route of elimination, because the eliminated drug enters the amniotic fluid, which is then swallowed by the fetus, in addition to which the drugs transferred to the fetus are eliminated more slowly than with the mother [10].

CHANGES IN THE URINARY TRACT DURING PREGNANCY

The urinary tract in the pregnant woman undergoes significant and important anatomical and physiological adaptive changes. These changes are summarized in Table **2** [22]. The renal length increases by approximately 1 cm and the glomerular filtration rate is increased by approximately 30% to 50%. Mild hydroureteronephrosis is observable as early as the seventh week of gestation. This dilatation is due to the general decrease in peristalsis in the collecting system and ureters, attributable to the myorelaxant effects of progesterone and progressive mechanical obstruction by the gravid uterus. During pregnancy, the bladder also experiences progressive anterior and upper displacement, as well as hypertrophy and gentle muscle relaxation, leading to increased urinary stasis and capacity [22].

Table 2. Urinary tract changes in Pregnancy [22].

Kidney	Increased renal length and glomerular filtration rate
Collecting System	Reduced peristalsis
Ureters	Reduced peristalsis, mechanical obstruction
Bladder	Displaced anteriorly and superiorly smooth muscle relaxation increased capacity

These changes increase the risk of developing pyelonephritis from asymptomatic bacteriuria (lower tract bacteriuria, cystitis) and urinary tract infections (UTIs) [22]. UTIs are the second most common pregnancy disease after anemia and, at the same time, the most common type of infection in pregnant women. It is estimated that 5-10% of pregnant women develop some type of UTI, which is the cause of approximately 5% of all hospital admissions [22, 23]. UTIs, even when asymptomatic, predispose to pyelonephritis, and may result in serious maternal and fetal complications such as: preterm labor, low birth weight or infections. Therefore, these infections represent considerable diagnostic and therapeutic challenges [22]. In summary, pregnancy significantly alters drug dynamics, with increased total body water rate and glomerular filtration, resulting in increased renal drug clearance, reduced distribution, altered protein binding, and changes in hepatic metabolism that may affect serum concentrations of the drug [3, 10].

CLASSIFICATION OF USED DRUGS IN PREGNANCY

Previously a classification system for drugs during pregnancy, published by the Food and Drug Administration (FDA), labeled them in classes A, B, C, D or X, according to the category of risk. In December 2014, the FDA approved a new pregnancy drug labeling system that would be more practical and help guide decision making by physicians and patients [24]. According to the new rules, the summary of characteristics of the medicinal product should contain information on the scope of use of a particular drug during pregnancy and on risks in pregnancy in the following four categories: structural, fetal and/or infant abnormalities, functional impairment, and changes in growth. The document should also report, where available, data on the risks of congenital anomalies and spontaneous abortions compared to their incidence in the general population, being vital and immediate sources of information for doctors [3].

Classification According to The Categories of Risk of Drugs in Pregnancy

The FDA put the new system into effect on June 30, 2015, for use in pregnancy. These categories were eliminated because most of the drugs were Category C, indicating a lack of data in humans. The designation of category C as opposed to B was distinctive for historical reasons. Because it is a recent change, the categories are maintained in the Table **3** for reference [25].

Table 3. Categories of drugs for use in pregnancy [25].

FDA Pregnancy Category	
Category A	Controlled studies do not demonstrate a risk to the fetus
Category B	Animal studies have shown adverse effect, but human studies show no risk
Category C	Animal studies have shown an adverse effect on the fetus and there are no controlled studies in humans
Category D	There is positive evidence of human fetal risk from investigational studies
Category X	Studies in animals or humans have demonstrated fetal abnormalities and/or there is positive evidence of human fetal risk based on adverse reaction data from investigational or marketing experience. The drug is contraindicated

Despite the lack of high-quality safety data, many antimicrobials have been used in pregnancy for years without adverse maternal or fetal outcomes, including penicillins, cephalosporins, clindamycin, and macrolides [25, 26].

ANTIBIOTICS AND OTHER ANTI-INFECTIOUS AGENTS IN PREGNANCY

Due to the physiological adaptations of pregnancy, vulvovaginal candidiasis and UTIs are more common and are associated with upper respiratory tract infections accounting for about 72% of all infections treated during pregnancy. For these reasons, antibiotics are the drugs most frequently used in pregnant women, accounting for approximately 80% of the medications administered [22, 23]. 5-10% of pregnant women develop asymptomatic bacteriuria during pregnancy, one third of cases will develop symptomatic UTIs with the potential to cause complications such as pyelonephritis, chorioamnionitis, premature rupture of membranes and preterm birth [26]. The WHO estimates that the overall prevalence of maternal infections is 4.4 per cent among live births, accounting for more than 5.7 million cases per year, it is considered a life-threatening condition and a leading direct cause of death worldwide, accounting for up to 10% of maternal deaths. The most common intervention to prevent morbidity and mortality related to maternal infection is the use of antibiotics for prophylaxis and treatment [2]. Penicillins make up 80% of antibiotic prescriptions during pregnancy and macrolides are the most frequent class. The most commonly used drugs, such as penicillins, cephalosporins and macrolides, have a long established safety record [26, 27].

Although widely used during pregnancy, antibiotics should be employed rationally because of their potential side effects, both for the mother and the fetus [2]. Must be used when indicated and there is benefit in their use. Clear recommendations are also made against the use of prophylactic antibiotics for all women with the aim of reducing infections during pregnancy or after an uncomplicated (or uninterrupted) vaginal delivery [2].

Betalactam and Related Antibiotics

Penicillins

Penicillins are the oldest known antibiotics [4]. They are derived from 6-aminopenicillanic acid and differ from each other depending on the substitution on the side chain of their amino group [20]. They act by inhibiting the synthesis of the cell wall of bacteria [28]. They belong to the β-lactam group and include aminopenicillins (amoxicillin and ampicillin), as well as flucloxacillin resistant to β-lactamase [29].

They are widely used against streptococcal, staphylococcal, enterococcal and meningococcal strains and are used in the treatment of syphilis, gonorrhea and meningitis [30]. It is known that penicillins can pass through the placental barrier and reach fetal blood and amniotic fluid at considerable levels, but there are no data on teratogenic therapeutic doses considered as first-line therapy in pregnancy. Moreover, their long-term security record is supported by the Birth Defects Prevention Study (NBDPS). However, resistance is a growing problem for ampicillin and maternal hypersensitivity is the main therapeutic restriction [31]. Topical penicillin can be used in pregnancy as they are classified in category B according to the FDA.

Several literatures have a reduction in serum penicillin levels, as well as an increase in renal clearance in the gestational period compared to the non-pregnant state. By means of simple diffusion, penicillins cross a placental barrier. Prescribing penicillins with weak protein binding, such as penicillin G, ampicillin and methicillin in the gestational period provides a greater concentration of drug slums in the fetal and amniotic fluid. In contrast, the use of penicillins with high protein binding, such as oxacillin, dicloxacillin, naphthylin and cloxacillin, promotes less bioavailability in fetal and amniotic fluid. The amniotic fluid will present antibiotics, derived from the excretion of fetal urine. After 60 minutes of intravenous administration, the concentration of penicillin G, ampicillin and methicillin in maternal serum and amniotic fluid are the same, ensuring rapid bioavailability for fetal circulation and amniotic fluid. During pregnancy it is essential to increase the dosage of penicillins, as most of them are excreted largely unchanged in the urine, with a small fraction that undergoes hepatic inactivation. To increase the spectrum of action, drugs can be associated with clavulanate, with no evidence of risks for birth defects [32]. For all penicillins and their derivatives, as well as for combinations of penicillins with β-lactamase inhibitors such as clavulanate or sulbactam, a category B classification has been assigned [5]. Pregnant patients with penicillin allergy diagnosed with syphilis should undergo desensitization followed by therapy with penicillin [5]. Oxacillin is a drug that is part of the group of penicillins resistant to beta-lactamase and staphylococcal penicillinase. Its main indication are for infections caused by these germs in various locations, namely abscesses, septicemia, pneumonia, *etc.*

Cephalosporins

Cephalosporins make up the group of B-lactams and have broad bactericidal activity, since they are resistant to B-lactamase and penicillinase. They are divided into five generations according to the spectrum of action and order of development.

The class includes second generation cefuroxime and first-generation cephalexin. Cephalosporins belong to category B and are used to treat various infections, such as: UTI, pneumonia, otitis and sinusitis, and severe bacterial infections [34]. NBDPS found a significant association only between cephalosporin and atrial septal defects [35]. However, to the authors' knowledge, this is the only study reporting this association, and NBDPS in general supports the long-established safety record of the use of cephalosporins in pregnancy [35]. Prospective studies on the use of cefuroxime and cephalexin in the first trimester did not find teratogenic or spontaneous abortion outcomes at the doses used. Cephalosporins may be considered generally safe for treatment during pregnancy. However, increased resistance to cephalosporins is a concern. Cephalosporins remain a first-line option for many infections in pregnancy with general use reserved for patients allergic or intolerant to therapy with penicillins [5]. In addition to cephalexin, cefazolin (first generation), cefuroxime axetil and cefuroxime (second generation), and cefriaxone (third generation) are the most commonly used. Ceftriaxone remains the drug of choice for the treatment of gonorrhea during pregnancy [5]. However, the use of these drugs confers a high risk of neonatal kernicterus (a disease that affects the brain tissue, excess of indirect bilirubin), therefore, its use should be considered. Recently approved agents such as ceftaroline, ceftolozane-tazobactam and ceftazidime-avibactam are also labeled as category B; however, they should be used with caution because of the lack of data during pregnancy that has been published [5].

When antibiotic treatment is required in the first trimester of pregnancy, antibiotics that have been used extensively (*e.g.*, penicillin, ampicillin, amoxicillin, and erythromycin) and which were not associated with an increased risk of congenital defects should be used in first-line therapy [41]. Maternal serum cephalosporin levels during pregnancy are lower than in non-pregnant patients receiving equivalent dosages due to a shorter half-life in pregnancy and an increase in the volume of distribution. Renal elimination is increased in pregnancy [41]. These drugs readily cross the placenta to the fetus, bloodstream, and finally the amniotic fluid [41].

Macrolides

Macrolides are drugs that bind to the bacterial ribosome and inhibit protein synthesis [36]. They are one of the most prescribed classes of antibiotics and are frequently used for infections of bacteria resistant to penicillin or in patients allergic to penicillin [36]. Macrolides are comprised of a large macrolactonic ring of 14 to 16 carbon atoms, to which one or more sugar molecules are attached. Since the discovery of the first macrolide, erythromycin, which is naturally produced by Saccharopolyspora erythraea, several second-generation macrolides with improved stability and efficacy, such as azithromycin, have been developed [36]. The main drugs belonging to this class are erythromycin, clarithromycin, azithromycin and spiramycin.

Erythromycin and its salts are not consistently absorbed by the gastrointestinal tract of pregnant women, and transplacental passage is unpredictable [37, 38]. Maternal and fetal serum levels achieved after drug administration in pregnancy are low and vary considerably, with fetal plasma concentrations of 5 to 20% of maternal plasma [37]. At high doses they may not be well tolerated in pregnant women, who are susceptible to nausea and gastrointestinal symptoms [32, 37]. Clarithromycin is a semisynthetic macrolide that aims to treat bacterial infections involving the skin, ear, paranasal sinuses and lungs, among others.

Azithromycin is an azalide, derived from erythromycin, with a nitrogen atom substituted by methyl incorporated into the lactone ring [38]. It binds to the 50S subunit of the bacterial ribosome and thus inhibits the translation of mRNA [38]. Azithromycin is used to treat or prevent certain bacterial infections, most often those that cause middle ear infections, throat infections, pneumonia, typhoid, bronchitis, and sinusitis [38]. Recently, it has been prescribed especially for the treatment of bacterial infections in neonates and immunosuppressed individuals. It is also effective in sexually transmitted infections such as non-gonococcal urethritis, chlamydia and cervicitis [38]. However, recent studies suggest there is a risk in the use of macrolides in pregnant women [33, 39].

Nitrofurans

Nitrofurantoin is an antimicrobial drug indicated for UTIs, with a view to its lower urinary tract preference in detriment to other tissues, as well as the fact that *E. coli*, the most frequent pathogen in urinary tract infection, is largely resistant to penicillin [40]. It is also endowed with antiprotozoal and antifungal activities. As asymptomatic bacteriuria is a condition of high prevalence during pregnancy, most medical guidelines support the treatment of this condition with this antibiotic. However, there is conflicting evidence about its use. Large population-based retrospective cohort studies report that quarterly exposure to nitrofurantoin was not associated with congenital malformations or spontaneous abortion [33, 40]. The excretion of nitrofurantoin is by renal route, in its active form, being particularly effective against *Escherichia coli*, *Enterococcus faecalis* and *Staphylococcus aureus*. The multiple forms of administration of nitrofurantoin explain the varying absorptions at the level of the gastrointestinal tract. The macrocrystalline form is absorbed more slowly than crystalline and is associated with less gastrointestinal intolerance, reducing adverse events such as nausea and vomiting, without, however, modifying its urinary concentration and its therapeutic action [41]. Therapeutic serum levels are not reached; therefore, this medication is not indicated when there is a possibility of bacteremia, as in pyelonephritis [32, 41]. Approximately one-third of an oral dose appears in the active form in the urine [41]. Compared to older antibiotics such as penicillin, trimethoprim-sulfamethoxazole and first-generation cephalosporins, nitrofurantoin demonstrates little or no bacterial resistance.

Aminoglycosides

Aminoglycosides include amikacin, streptomycin, gentamycin, neomycin, kanamycin, ribostamycin and tobramycin. The name aminoglycoside is due to the fact that the molecule consists of two or more amino sugars linked by glycosidic attachment to the hexose or aminocyclitol, which is usually in a central position [42]. Its antimicrobial activity occurs mainly in alkaline and aerobic pH medium, a necessary condition to carry out the transport of substances through the plasma membrane (active transport). The pharmacokinetics of all aminoglycosides are quite similar [42]. Due to their polar nature, they are poorly absorbed by the gastrointestinal tract, with less than 1% of the dose being absorbed after oral or rectal administration [42]. The main route of administration is therefore parenteral, with the drug reaching peak plasma concentration after 30-90 minutes of intramuscular application [42]. Excluding streptomycin, which is around 30% bound to albumin, the other aminoglycosides have only 10% protein binding. The fact that they are insoluble in lipids causes their concentration in secretions and in tissues to be reduced, since they inefficiently cross the biological membranes that do not have a transport mechanism [42]. The half-life of the blood is two to three hours in patients with normal renal function [42]. Renal excretion is the mechanism for eliminating these drugs, and clearance is about 66% of simultaneous creatinine clearance, which is a function of tubular reabsorption. The half-life in the renal cortex is estimated to be between 30-700 hours, which means that there is still urinary elimination 20 to 30 days after administration of the last dose of the drug [42]. All aminoglycosides act by the same mechanism of action, exerting their bactericidal effect when binding to the bacterial ribosome [42]. Among the aminoglycosides with a potential risk of deafness and ototoxicity in newborns are gentamicin, streptomycin and kanamycin. Its use within the first 4 months of pregnancy is not recommended unless there is no alternative available. However, there is a growing body of evidence to support its use in pregnancy. A large epidemiological study did not link aminoglycosides to ototoxicity and parenteral gentamicin, while oral neomycin and other aminoglycosides were not associated with an increased rate of congenital diseases [18]. Gentamicin is the preferred aminoglycoside and has a more reliable safety record, several scientific tests have proven its safety and effectiveness in cases of endometritis and chorioamnionitis. It is commonly used in obstetrics and gynecology for UTI, but more evidence is needed to support the use of ribostamycin and tobramycin in pregnancy [18]. It was found that the combination of aminoglycosides and cephalosporins caused nephrotoxicity, and therefore should be avoided [18].

Lincosamides

Clindamycin

Clindamycin is a lincosamide antibiotic with macrolide-like applications. It has a high efficacy against anaerobes and gram-positive bacteria and is prescribed to treat of bacterial vaginosis if treatment is given early in pregnancy and for patients with penicillin hypersensitivity [29]. It inhibits bacterial protein synthesis and, depending on its concentration and sensitivity, can be bactericidal or bacteriostatic. Its use is indicated when penicillins, cephalosporins and macrolides fail [5]. Clindamycin crosses the placenta reaching serum levels in the umbilical cord of around 50% of that of maternal serum. Evidence strongly supports the safe use of clindamycin during pregnancy and there are no known teratogenic effects when used topically or orally. In contrast, vaginal administration is not recommended because of systemic absorption (up to 30%), increased risk of adverse neonatal outcomes (neonatal infection and low birth weight) and ineffectiveness [43]. Late use of clindamycin until the 32nd week of gestation is associated with adverse outcomes. Thus, the Centers for Disease Control and Prevention of Sexually Transmitted Diseases Treatment Guidelines recommend avoiding vaginal clindamycin in the second half of pregnancy [5, 43]. Most of the drug is metabolized in the liver into products excreted in urine and bile, and only 10% of the drug is excreted unchanged in the urine [41, 42].

Quinolones

Quinolones, which include for example ciprofloxacin and levofloxacin, is a group of antibiotics that inhibits bacterial enzymes topoisomerase II and IV, which are important for the metabolism of nucleic acids [5]. They reach high tissue concentrations, thus making them an effective choice for pyelonephritis in non-pregnant patients, but are generally avoided during pregnancy because of possible arthropathies and teratogenicity, since they have a high affinity for cartilage and bone tissue, which is higher in immature cartilage, as it can cross the placenta and be found in amniotic fluid in low concentrations [1, 5, 18]. In animal models, it has been observed that quinolones can induce abnormalities in the development of cartilaginous tissue [1]. Interestingly, when pregnant women were exposed to quinolones, adverse events were not consistently demonstrated. In general, this class of antimicrobials should be avoided in pregnancy if other suitable alternatives are available [1, 29]. In challenging situations, when better studied antibiotics are ineffective, well documented quinolones may be preferred, such as norfloxacin or ciprofloxacin [5]. A detailed ultrasound examination should be performed after exposure with other fluoroquinolones during the first trimester [5].

Antifungals with Application in Pregnancy

Metronidazole

Metronidazole acts by inhibiting DNA synthesis and is prescribed in cases of anaerobic and protozoal infections. It can be given orally or locally. Several studies have recommended its use during pregnancy for the prevention of preterm birth in the treatment of bacterial vaginosis [5, 44]. Metronidazole topical (category B) is minimally absorbed and considered safe in pregnancy. Relatively high concentrations may reach the fetus when administered orally. When administered intravenously or orally at the usual recommended doses, metronidazole reaches concentrations well above the minimum inhibitory concentrations for the most susceptible microorganisms [28]. Its parenteral administration is indicated for severe infections only [5]. The drug has an oral bioavailability approaching 100% [28]. Rectal and vaginal administration results in less drug absorption and lower serum concentration [28]. Metronidazole has limited binding to plasma proteins, but can achieve very favorable tissue distribution, including in the CNS [45]. The drug is extensively metabolized in the liver to form two primary oxidative metabolites: the hydroxy and acetic acid metabolites [45]. The kidney is responsible for eliminating only a small amount of the original medicine [45]. Metronidazole is generally well tolerated when given in doses <2g per day [28]. Some adverse reactions, such as gastrointestinal effects, neuropathies and certain effects on the central nervous system, appear to be related to dosage and duration of treatment [28, 46, 47]. Although this medication has a mutagenic and carcinogenic potential evidenced experimentally in the laboratory, long-standing studies and investigations have not shown the teratogenic potential of metronidazole in humans [5].

Clotrimazole

All azole antifungal drugs interfere with the biosynthesis of ergosterol, which is an important component of the fungal cytoplasmic membrane. Specifically, azole including clotrimazole inhibits the demethylation of the cytochrome P450 (CYP450], which is a vital step in fungus ergosterol biosynthesis. Depletion of ergosterol and its substitution by the aberrant species of the sterol, 14- α-methylsterol, disrupt the normal permeability and fluidity of the membrane.

Clotrimazole is used in the treatment of tinea pedis, tinea cruris, tinea corporis and cutaneous candidiasis [48]. 0.5% of the dose applied topically is absorbed systemically [48]. Topical clotrimazole is safe in pregnancy, and some authors consider it a first-line topical drug for cutaneous mycoses, being especially strongly indicated for the treatment of external genital infections and adjacent areas in women, as well as in their sexual partner, caused by yeasts [48, 49]. Studies in animals with high doses did not cause teratogenicity, however, its use in the first 3 months of pregnancy should be recommended only after careful medical evaluation, with the treatment performed using only a single dose vaginal tablet, which should be inserted without the use of the applicator [50]. There are studies that question the use of clotrimazole to prevent premature birth in women with asymptomatic candidiasis, resulting in screening protocols that are directly implicated in the management of pregnant women and may be readily incorporated into routine prenatal care with reduced premature births [51].

Miconazole

Miconazole, along with clotrimazole, is a well-investigated local antifungal for use in pregnancy. Its systemic absorption is insignificant, and for this reason it is considered safe, and may represent a first-line topical therapy for fungal infections [48, 49]. Data from the Michigan Medicaid program, where 2236 women and 7266 newborns were exposed to miconazole during the first trimester, showed that there was no connection between miconazole and congenital, cardiovascular, orthopedic, spina bifida, polydactyly, limb reduction defects or hypospadias [48, 49]. Although there is a study showing a link between vaginal miconazole therapies associated with metronidazole during the second and third months and an increase in the appearance of syndactyly and hexadactyly, this theory has not been confirmed by other researchers [5]. Thus, miconazole and clotrimazole should, whenever possible, be the preferred drugs for the topical treatment of fungal infections during pregnancy [5].

Antivirals

Acyclovir

Acyclovir is indicated for herpes simplex virus (HSV) infections [48]. Topical acyclovir is minimally absorbed systemically [48]. Animal and human studies using aciclovir did not report adverse fetal outcomes [48]. In a Danish study of 1031 women, topical acyclovir use 1-4 weeks before conception, in 2850 women in the 1st trimester and in 5447 women in the 2nd and 3rd trimesters, did not present major congenital defects in relation to the non-exposed group [48]. One drug manufacturer was aware of the topical use of acyclovir in two pregnant patients during the third trimester [48]. Although both had normal babies, these cases remain unpublished [48]. Topical acyclovir is considered safe for use in pregnancy [49, 52]. Additional studies that investigated the efficacy of this drug for viral suppression in the advanced stage of pregnancy (> 36 weeks) did not show evidence of adverse effects in neonates [53]. The Aciclovir Registry recorded 601 exposures during pregnancy, including 425 in the first trimester, with no increased risk of abnormalities in infants [41]. Maternal systemic acyclovir has also been used in the short term to prevent recurrent genital herpes without adverse effects in infants [41]. The Centers for Disease Control and Prevention recommends that pregnant women with disseminated infection, *e.g.*, herpetic encephalitis or hepatitis or varicella pneumonia, should be treated with acyclovir [32].

Penciclovir

Penciclovir is indicated for the treatment of recurrent herpes simplex [48]. A study indicated that plasma concentration after a 1% topical dose application was undetectable [54]. Animal studies using oral penciclovir, at 260 and 355 times the maximum recommended dose, did not report adverse fetal outcomes [48]. In a Danish study, 34 women exposed to penciclovir 1-4 weeks before conception, 118 women in the first trimester and 206 women in the 2nd and 3rd trimesters, did not present increased congenital defects compared to the non-exposed group [48]. The study did not draw firm conclusions about the safety of penciclovir because of the small sample size [48]. After first-line medications, such as acyclovir, the use of topical penciclovir is permitted [48, 49].

Trichloroacetic Acid (TCA)

TCA is used to treat anogenital warts. Topical application results in insignificant systemic absorption and produces no systemic effects [48]. A study with 32 women treated with carbon dioxide laser therapy and 85% TCA did not report adverse perinatal outcomes [48]. Many consider TCA safe to use during pregnancy and recommend it as first-line therapy, or second line after cryotherapy for warts [48, 49]. The use of this antiviral in the second half of pregnancy is associated with higher clearance rates and a lower number of recurrences [55].

Short lesions have a better response to the drug, as they favor its penetration and the chemical coagulation process of wart protein, mechanism responsible for eliminating the lesion. On the other hand, in large and bulky lesions, TCA may not penetrate all verrucous tissue and, therefore, not generate the expected response to treatment.

Zidovudine/Lamivudine/Nevirapine

For obvious reasons, the drugs zidovudine, lamivudine and neviraprine are grouped together in this topic for their combined application as 1st line therapy for HIV infections. Although the administration of antiretrovirals is becoming more frequent in pregnant women, there is a lack of data on the consequences on fetal development. In contrast, the use of antiretroviral agents dramatically reduces the risk of vertical transmission [56, 57]. Combination antiretroviral therapy has been the most effective against HIV virus (control of viral load) and improved immune response in terms of CD4 cell count [55]. The scheme comprises combining at least three different antiretroviral drugs of at least two classes, such as:

1. Combination of two nucleotides reverse transcriptase inhibitors (NRTIs) including nucleoside reverse transcriptase inhibitors (NtRTIs),

2. Combination of two NRTIs including a protease inhibitor (PI),

3. Combination of two NRTIs including one PI plus one non-nucleotide reverse transcriptase inhibitor (NNRTI) or others [55].

Although antiretroviral therapy was not able to fully cure the disease, the combination regimen definitely helped reduce morbidity and mortality rates among HIV-infected patients [55, 58].

Combined antiretroviral regimens used in pregnancy should, where possible, contain zidovudine and lamivudine associated with nelfinavir or nevirapine. The choice between nelfinavir and nevirapine should consider the gestational age, the degree of maternal immunodeficiency, the magnitude of the viral load, the potential adherence to clinical follow-up and medication use. Nelfinavir is mostly indicated for gestational ages below 28 weeks and for women with more severe immunosuppression. Nevirapine should only be used in triple therapy, since its administration as a monotherapy implies the development of viral resistance of a significant proportion [59].

CONCLUSIONS

The use of anti-infective agents in pregnant women remains a challenge [43]. There is limited understanding of the altered pharmacokinetics of anti-infectives in this population, and as a result, optimized dosing regimens still need to be established [43]. Recent studies on pharmacology in pregnancy highlight the complexity of drug delivery and response in light of the dynamic gestational process [10]. Extrapolating drug dosage and expected responses from non-pregnant populations are inappropriate and may result in iatrogenic illness [10]. Instead, a structured approach to the pharmacokinetic and pharmacodynamic properties of the drugs used in pregnancy should be the focus [10]. In the absence of drug-specific data, rigorous patient monitoring is the most logical step in optimizing drug therapy in pregnant patients [10]. It should be noted that the complexity of the topic in the face of the current challenge of developing resistance to infectious agents is due to the indiscriminate use of drugs. Health professionals should consider the teratogenic and toxic risk profiles of anti-infective agents while making appropriate prescribing decisions.

CONSENT FOR PUBLICATION

Not applicable.

CONFLICT OF INTEREST

The authors declare no conflict of interest, financial or otherwise.

ACKNOWLEDGEMENTS

Declared none.

REFERENCES

[1]   Bonet M, Oladapo OT, Khan DN, Mathai M, Gülmezoglu AM. New WHO guidance on prevention and treatment of maternal peripartum infections. Lancet Glob Health 2015; 3(11): e667-8.
[http://dx.doi.org/10.1016/S2214-109X(15)00213-2] [PMID: 26429594]

[2]   Bonet M. Frequency and management of maternal infection in health facilities in 52 countries (GLOSS): a 1-week inception cohort study. Lancet Glob Health 2020; 8(5): e661-71.
[http://dx.doi.org/10.1016/S2214-109X(20)30109-1] [PMID: 32353314]

[3]   Sachdeva P, Patel BG, Patel BK. Drug use in pregnancy; a point to ponder! Indian J Pharm Sci 2009; 71(1): 1-7.
[http://dx.doi.org/10.4103/0250-474X.51941] [PMID: 20177448]

[4]   Baños JE. Use of antibiotics in pregnant patients in the intensive care unit. Infectious Diseases in Critical Care 2007.

[5]   Padberg S. Anti-infective Agents. Drugs During Pregnancy and Lactation 2015; pp. 115-76.

[6]   Gwee A, Cranswick N. Anti-infective use in children and pregnancy: current deficiencies and future challenges. Br J Clin Pharmacol 2015; 79(2): 216-21.

[http://dx.doi.org/10.1111/bcp.12363] [PMID: 24588467]

[7]   Rao GA, Mann JR, Shoaibi A, *et al.* Azithromycin and levofloxacin use and increased risk of cardiac arrhythmia and death. Ann Fam Med 2014; 12(2): 121-7.
[http://dx.doi.org/10.1370/afm.1601] [PMID: 24615307]

[8]   Piola P, Nabasumba C, Turyakira E, *et al.* Efficacy and safety of artemether-lumefantrine compared with quinine in pregnant women with uncomplicated *Plasmodium falciparum* malaria: an open-label, randomised, non-inferiority trial. Lancet Infect Dis 2010; 10(11): 762-9.
[http://dx.doi.org/10.1016/S1473-3099(10)70202-4] [PMID: 20932805]

[9]   Waller DG, Sampson AP. Waller, Anthony P Sampson "Pharmacokinetics. Elsevier BV 2018.

[10] Feghali M, Venkataramanan R, Caritis S. Pharmacokinetics of drugs in pregnancy. Semin Perinatol 2015; 39(7): 512-9.
[http://dx.doi.org/10.1053/j.semperi.2015.08.003] [PMID: 26452316]

[11] Ansari J, Carvalho B, Shafer SL, Flood P. Pharmacokinetics and pharmacodynamics of drugs commonly used in pregnancy and parturition. Anesth Analg 2016; 122(3): 786-804.
[http://dx.doi.org/10.1213/ANE.0000000000001143] [PMID: 26891392]

[12] Patil AS, Sheng JS, Dotters-Katz SK, Schmoll MS, Onslow ML. Principles of anti-infective dosing in pregnancy. Clin Ther 2016; 38(9): 2006-15.
[http://dx.doi.org/10.1016/j.clinthera.2016.08.005] [PMID: 27614913]

[13] Mitchell AA, Gilboa SM, Werler MM, Kelley KE, Louik C, Hernández-Díaz S. Medication use during pregnancy, with particular focus on prescription drugs: 1976-2008. Am J Obstet Gynecol 2011; 205(1): 51.e1-8.
[http://dx.doi.org/10.1016/j.ajog.2011.02.029] [PMID: 21514558]

[14] Moniz MH, Beigi RH. Vaccination during Pregnancy. Obstet Gynecol Surv 2016; 71(3): 178-86.
[http://dx.doi.org/10.1097/OGX.0000000000000283] [PMID: 26987582]

[15] Buxton ILO. Pharmacokinetics: The dynamics of drug absorption, distribution, metabolism, and elimination.Goodman & Gilman: The Pharmacological Basis of Therapeutics. 13th ed. New York: McGraw-Hill 2018; pp. 13-29.

[16] Costantine MM. Physiologic and pharmacokinetic changes in pregnancy. Front Pharmacol 2014; 5: 65.
[http://dx.doi.org/10.3389/fphar.2014.00065] [PMID: 24772083]

[17] Dallmann A. Gestation-specific changes in the anatomy and physiology of healthy pregnant women: An extended repository of model parameters for physiologically based pharmacokinetic modeling in pregnancy. Clin Pharmacokinet 2017; 56(11): 1303-30.
[http://dx.doi.org/10.1007/s40262-017-0539-z] [PMID: 28401479]

[18] Mannucci C, Dante G, Miroddi M, Facchinetti F, *et al.* Vigilance on use of drugs, herbal products, and food supplements during pregnancy: focus on fosfomycin. J Matern Fetal Neonatal Med 2018; 32(1): 125-8.
[PMID: 28868940]

[19] Nahum GG, Uhl K, Kennedy DL. Antibiotic use in pregnancy and lactation: what is and is not known about teratogenic and toxic risks. Obstet Gynecol 2006; 107(5): 1120-38.
[http://dx.doi.org/10.1097/01.AOG.0000216197.26783.b5] [PMID: 16648419]

[20] Institute of Medicine (US) Committee on the Ethical and Legal Issues Relating to the Inclusion of Women in Clinical Studies. 1999. https://www.ncbi.nlm.nih.gov/books/NBK236568/

[21] Jancova P, Anzenbacher P, Anzenbacherova E. Phase II drug metabolizing enzymes. Biomed Pap Med Fac Univ Palacky Olomouc Czech Repub 2010; 154(2): 103-16.
[http://dx.doi.org/10.5507/bp.2010.017] [PMID: 20668491]

[22] Glaser AP, Schaeffer AJ. Urinary tract infection and bacteriuria in pregnancy. Urol Clin North Am

2015; 42(4): 547-60.
[http://dx.doi.org/10.1016/j.ucl.2015.05.004] [PMID: 26475951]

[23]   Szweda H, Jóźwik M. Urinary tract infections during pregnancy - an updated overview. Dev Period Med 2016; 20(4): 263-72.
[PMID: 28216479]

[24]   FDA. FDA. Content and format of labeling for human prescription drug and biological products; requirements for pregnancy and lactation labeling. Fed Regist 2014; 79(233): 103-72063.

[25]   Khalid A. Drugs use or abuse; pharmacological considerations. Am J Biomed Sci & Res 2019; 5(3)

[26]   Lamont HF, Blogg HJ, Lamont RF. Safety of antimicrobial treatment during pregnancy: a current review of resistance, immunomodulation and teratogenicity. Expert Opin Drug Saf 2014; 13(12): 1569-81.
[http://dx.doi.org/10.1517/14740338.2014.939580] [PMID: 25189188]

[27]   Miller EL. The penicillins: a review and update. J Midwifery Womens Health 2002; 47(6): 426-34.
[http://dx.doi.org/10.1016/S1526-9523(02)00330-6] [PMID: 12484664]

[28]   Hernández M, Borrull F, Calull M. Analysis of antibiotics in biological samples by capillary electrophoresis. Trends Analyt Chem 2003; 22(7): 416-27.
[http://dx.doi.org/10.1016/S0165-9936(03)00702-7]

[29]   Wintermans BB, Vandenbroucke-Grauls CM. Outline of a bacterial filter-based assay to detect beta-lactamases. J Microbiol Methods 2016; 120: 29-33.
[http://dx.doi.org/10.1016/j.mimet.2015.11.013] [PMID: 26602625]

[30]   Katanami Y, Hashimoto T, Takaya S, et al. Amoxicillin and ceftriaxone as treatment alternatives to penicillin for maternal syphilis. Emerg Infect Dis 2017; 23(5): 827-9.
[http://dx.doi.org/10.3201/eid2305.161936] [PMID: 28418316]

[31]   Bizzarro MJ, Dembry LM, Baltimore RS, Gallagher PG. Changing patterns in neonatal Escherichia coli sepsis and ampicillin resistance in the era of intrapartum antibiotic prophylaxis. Pediatrics 2008; 121(4): 689-96.
[http://dx.doi.org/10.1542/peds.2007-2171] [PMID: 18381532]

[32]   Niebyl JR. Antibiotics and other anti-infective agents in pregnancy and lactation. Am J Perinatol 2003; 20(8): 405-14.
[http://dx.doi.org/10.1055/s-2003-45391] [PMID: 14703588]

[33]   Muanda FT, Sheehy O, Bérard A. Use of antibiotics during pregnancy and the risk of major congenital malformations: a population based cohort study. Br J Clin Pharmacol 2017; 83(11): 2557-71.
[http://dx.doi.org/10.1111/bcp.13364] [PMID: 28722171]

[34]   Thorpe PG, Gilboa SM, Hernandez-Diaz S, et al. Medications in the first trimester of pregnancy: most common exposures and critical gaps in understanding fetal risk. Pharmacoepidemiol Drug Saf 2013; 22(9): 1013-8.
[http://dx.doi.org/10.1002/pds.3495] [PMID: 23893932]

[35]   Archabald KL, Friedman A, Raker CA, Anderson BL. Impact of trimester on morbidity of acute pyelonephritis in pregnancy. Am J Obstet Gynecol 2009; 201(4): 406.e1-4.
[http://dx.doi.org/10.1016/j.ajog.2009.06.067] [PMID: 19691948]

[36]   Pavlova A, Parks JM, Oyelere AK, Gumbart JC. Toward the rational design of macrolide antibiotics to combat resistance. Chem Biol Drug Des 2017; 90(5): 641-52.
[http://dx.doi.org/10.1111/cbdd.13004] [PMID: 28419786]

[37]   Philipson A, Sabath LD, Charles D. Transplacental passage of erythromycin and clindamycin. N Engl J Med 1973; 288(23): 1219-21.
[http://dx.doi.org/10.1056/NEJM197306072882307] [PMID: 4700555]

[38]   Bakheit AH, Al-Hadiya BM, Abd-Elgalil AA. Azithromycin. Profiles Drug Subst Excip Relat

Methodol 2014; 39: 1-40.
[http://dx.doi.org/10.1016/B978-0-12-800173-8.00001-5] [PMID: 24794904]

[39]   Muanda FT, Sheehy O, Bérard A. Use of antibiotics during pregnancy and risk of spontaneous abortion. CMAJ 2017; 189(17): E625-33.
[http://dx.doi.org/10.1503/cmaj.161020] [PMID: 28461374]

[40]   Goldberg O. Exposure to nitrofurantoin during early pregnancy and congenital malformations: A systematic review and meta-analysis. J Obstet Gynaecol Can 2015; 37(2): 6-150.

[41]   Munoz-Davila MJ. Role of old antibiotics in the era of antibiotic resistance. highlighted nitrofurantoin for the treatment of lower urinary tract infections. Antibiotics (Basel) 2014; 3(1): 39-48.
[http://dx.doi.org/10.3390/antibiotics3010039] [PMID: 27025732]

[42]   Oliveira JFP, Cipullo JP II, Burdmann EA III. Aminoglycoside nephrotoxicity. Rev Bras Cir Cardiovasc 2006; 21(4): 444-52.
[http://dx.doi.org/10.1590/S0102-76382006000400015]

[43]   Bookstaver PB, Bland CM, Griffin B, Stover KR, Eiland LS, McLaughlin M. A review of antibiotic use in pregnancy. Pharmacotherapy 2015; 35(11): 1052-62.
[http://dx.doi.org/10.1002/phar.1649] [PMID: 26598097]

[44]   Koss CA, Baras DC, Lane SD, *et al.* Investigation of metronidazole use during pregnancy and adverse birth outcomes. Antimicrob Agents Chemother 2012; 56(9): 4800-5.
[http://dx.doi.org/10.1128/AAC.06477-11] [PMID: 22751543]

[45]   Lau AH, Lam NP, Piscitelli SC, Wilkes L, Danziger LH. Clinical pharmacokinetics of metronidazole and other nitroimidazole anti-infectives. Clin Pharmacokinet 1992; 23(5): 328-64.
[http://dx.doi.org/10.2165/00003088-199223050-00002] [PMID: 1478003]

[46]   Agarwal A, Kanekar S, Sabat S, Thamburaj K. Metronidazole-induced cerebellar toxicity. Neurol Int 2016; 8(1): 6365.
[http://dx.doi.org/10.4081/ni.2016.6365] [PMID: 27127600]

[47]   Lewis BB, Buffie CG, Carter RA, *et al.* Loss of microbiota-mediated colonization resistance to clostridium difficile infection with oral vancomycin compared with metronidazole. J Infect Dis 2015; 212(10): 1656-65.
[http://dx.doi.org/10.1093/infdis/jiv256] [PMID: 25920320]

[48]   Patil AS, Sheng J, Dotters-Katz SK, Schmoll MS, Onslow M, Pierson RC. Fundamentals of clinical pharmacology with application for pregnant women. J Midwifery Womens Health 2017; 62(3): 298-307.
[http://dx.doi.org/10.1111/jmwh.12621] [PMID: 28498553]

[49]   Patel VM, Schwartz RA, Lambert WC. Topical antiviral and antifungal medications in pregnancy: a review of safety profiles. J Eur Acad Dermatol Venereol 2017; 31(9): 1440-6.
[http://dx.doi.org/10.1111/jdv.14297] [PMID: 28449377]

[50]   Crowley PD, Gallagher HC. Clotrimazole as a pharmaceutical: past, present and future. J Appl Microbiol 2014; 117(3): 611-7.
[http://dx.doi.org/10.1111/jam.12554] [PMID: 24863842]

[51]   Roberts CL, Rickard K, Kotsiou G, Morris JM. Treatment of asymptomatic vaginal candidiasis in pregnancy to prevent preterm birth: an open-label pilot randomized controlled trial. BMC Pregnancy Childbirth 2011; 11: 18.
[http://dx.doi.org/10.1186/1471-2393-11-18] [PMID: 21396090]

[52]   Pasternak B, Hviid A. Use of acyclovir, valacyclovir, and famciclovir in the first trimester of pregnancy and the risk of birth defects. JAMA 2010; 304(8): 859-66.
[http://dx.doi.org/10.1001/jama.2010.1206] [PMID: 20736469]

[53]   Cottreau JM, Barr VO. A review of antiviral and antifungal use and safety during pregnancy. Pharmacotherapy 2016; 36(6): 668-78.

[http://dx.doi.org/10.1002/phar.1764] [PMID: 27139037]

[54]   Murase JE, Heller MM, Butler DC. Safety of dermatologic medications in pregnancy and lactation: Part I. Pregnancy. J Am Acad Dermatol 2014; 70(3): 401.e1-401.e14.
[http://dx.doi.org/10.1016/j.jaad.2013.09.010] [PMID: 24528911]

[55]   Feghali M, Venkataramanan R, Caritis S. Pharmacokinetics of drugs in pregnancy. Semin Perinatol. 2015; 39: pp. (7)512-9.
[http://dx.doi.org/10.1053/j.semperi.2015.08.003]

[56]   Zhang Z, Unadkat JD. Development of a novel maternal-fetal physiologically based pharmacokinetic model II: Verification of the model for passive placental permeability drugs. Drug Metab Dispos 2017; 45(8): 939-46.
[http://dx.doi.org/10.1124/dmd.116.073957] [PMID: 28049636]

[57]   Rough K, Sun JW, Seage GR III, *et al.* Zidovudine use in pregnancy and congenital malformations. AIDS 2017; 31(12): 1733-43.
[http://dx.doi.org/10.1097/QAD.0000000000001549] [PMID: 28537936]

[58]   Joshi A, Gbadero D, Esseku F, Adesanya OJ, Adeyeye MC. A randomized two-way crossover bioequivalence study in healthy adult volunteers of paediatric zidovudine/lamivudine/nevirapine fast-disintegrating fixed-dose combination tablet. J Pharm Pharmacol 2017; 69(4): 463-70.
[http://dx.doi.org/10.1111/jphp.12666] [PMID: 27859251]

[59]   Samuel R, Julian MN, Paredes R, *et al.* HIV-1 drug resistance by ultra-deep sequencing following short course zidovudine, single-dose nevirapine, and single-dose tenofovir with emtricitabine for prevention of mother-to-child transmission. J Acquir Immune Defic Syndr 2016; 73(4): 384-9.
[http://dx.doi.org/10.1097/QAI.0000000000001116] [PMID: 27327263]

CHAPTER 3

Classification and Safety of Anti-Infective Agents During Pregnancy

Jaline de Melo Pessoa Cavalcante[1], Fernanda Coêlho Paiva[1], Janaína Crispim Freitas[2], Diana Gonçalves Dantas[1], Luana Paiva Souza[1] and Ricardo Ney Cobucci[1]

[1] *Medicine School and Biotechnology Postgraduate Program, Potiguar University-UnP, Salgado Filho Av., 1610, Natal - RN, Zip code 59056-000, Brazil*

[2] *Women Health Postgraduate Program and Pharmacy Department, Federal University of Rio Grande do Norte, Natal, Brazil*

Abstract: The use of medication during pregnancy represents a challenge for health professionals, since the incorrect use leads to harmful effects not only on the pregnant woman but also on the fetus. Most anti-infective agents administered to pregnant women cross the placental barrier and expose the developing fetus to their pharmacological effects, which may be teratogenic. Because of the relatively common occurrence of some infections during pregnancy, there is a great importance of studying them, therefore, knowing the classification of the drugs and identifying which agents are safe during pregnancy will both be discussed in this chapter.

Keywords: Aminoglycosides, Antifungals, Antiviral agents, Antimalarial agents, Antihelminticos, Betalactams, Chloramphenicol, Lincosamides, Macrolides, Metronidazole, Nitrofurantoin, Quinolones, Rifampicin, Sulfonamides, Tetracyclines.

BACKGROUND

According to the Food and Drug Administration (FDA), most women take at least one medication during pregnancy, which often cannot be interrupted because it is part of a previously used therapy, such as treatments for asthma, hypertension, depression and diabetes mellitus [1]. In addition, the state of pregnancy causes physiological changes in women, affecting the way the medication is absorbed, metabolized and eliminated by the body [2].

* **Corresponding author Ricardo Ney Cobucci:** Medicine School and Biotechnology Postgraduate Program, Potiguar University-UnP, Salgado Filho Av., 1610, Natal - RN, Zip code 59056-000, Brazil; Tel: +5584 3215 1234; E-mail: rncobucci@hotmail.com

Therefore, in order to better understand the risk and safety of medicines, the FDA in 1979 developed a classification system based on five categories (A, B, C, D and X), which considered risks of medicines during pregnancy, mainly the first trimester, based on human and animal studies [1, 3]:

- Category A - studies on women who did not show any risk to the fetus during the first trimester (REMOTE FETAL DAMAGE);

- Category B - animal studies that did not indicate risk to the fetus, but there are no studies on women which can prove so (CAUTION);

- Category C - animal studies have demonstrated teratogenic or toxic effects on the fetus, however, there are no controlled studies on pregnant women or there are no controlled studies on animals or humans (RISKY);

- Category D - there is evidence of risk for fetuses, but the benefits for the pregnant woman may be acceptable (HIGH RISK);

- Category X - animal or human studies have shown that the drug causes fetal changes or that there is evidence of increased risk for the fetus based on experience in humans or both. The risk is clearly greater than any potential benefit (DANGER).

However, the FDA received comments on how categories were not very clear, resulting in misinterpretation and false assumptions about the real meaning of each of them. In addition, the risks of drugs in breastfeeding and possible general adverse effects were not taken into account.

For this reason, in 2015, the FDA decided to change the classification and developed the Pregnancy and Lactation Labeling Rule (PLLR or final rule), whose main objective is to expose drug information with greater clarity to assist decision making by both the physician and the patient. This new system requires that the labeling must include a summary of the risks of using a drug during pregnancy and lactation, a discussion on the data supporting this summary and relevant information for prescribers and pregnant women [3].

Although the PLLR is more complete than the first classification, it still does not provide a definitive answer whether the drug is safe to use during pregnancy and, therefore, individualizing each case is still essential when taking decisions. Although the new rule is already used, some drugs continue to be classified in the old way. Therefore, in this chapter, we have addressed both rules for a more in-depth and complete understanding of all the information that is essential when prescribing a drug during pregnancy.

ANTIMICROBIALS

Penicillins

Penicillins are the most frequently prescribed antibiotic group in the beta-lactams class. The main function is to inhibit the growth of sensitive bacteria by inactivating enzymes located on the bacterial cell membrane, conferring a bactericidal action [2, 4, 5].

This class can be classified into three categories, however, in pregnant women, only two types can be used: penicillin G and broad-spectrum penicillins. Benzathine penicillin G is classified as category B, according to the FDA. This antibiotic is indicated for the treatment of: pneumococcal infections (*Pneumococcus spp*), such as moderately severe pneumonia and otitis media; group A streptococcal infections not associated to bacteremia, upper respiratory tract, scarlet fever, erysipelas, skin and soft tissue infections and syphilitic infections (*Treponema pallidum*). In addition, it can be used to prevent rheumatic fever [6, 7].

In pregnant women, it is the first option in the treatment of syphilis [8]. Parenteral (intramuscular) penicillin G is the only treatment with proven safety and efficacy for the mother and fetus throughout pregnancy. Pregnant women with a history of allergy to penicillin should be desensitized and subsequently treated with penicillin [6].

Among the adverse effects of penicillin G, we emphasize anaphylactic reactions/hypersensitivity, fibrosis and atrophy, methemoglobinemia, superinfection (including diarrhea associated with *Clostridium* due to difficulties and pseudomembranous colitis) in pregnant women [7]. As this drug is present in milk, there may be changes in the intestinal flora of infants and, therefore, these individuals should be monitored for gastrointestinal disorders, such as diarrhea and thrush [8].

Broad-spectrum penicillins are active against gram-negative bacilli. Among the penicillins belonging to this group, amoxicillin, category B by the FDA, can be used for pregnant women as an alternative treatment for Chlamydia [9]. This antibiotic is active against most strains of *Escherichia coli*, *Proteus mirabilis*, *Salmonella*, *Shigella* and *Haemophilus influenzae* [4].

Ampicillin, classified as category B by the FDA, is a member of the broad spectrum penicillin group and belongs to aminopenicillins [3]. It is of great importance in the treatment of community-acquired pneumonia, otitis media, acute bacterial rhinosinusitis, skin and soft tissue infections, group A streptococcal cariango tonsillitis, and urinary tract infections [7, 10].

In pregnant women, its use is recommended in cases of premature rupture of membranes (PROM) and women who will go through normal birth and are classified as high risk for endocarditis. In neonates, it is used to prevent infections by group B Streptococcus (GBS) [11].

From pharmacological aspects, it achieves a fetal concentration equal to the maternal concentration, concentration in the amniotic fluid equal to or greater than the maternal one, and therefore this drug has an effective therapeutic level, with no harmful effects to the fetus reported. In addition, as it is present in breast milk, it should be administered with caution to women who are breastfeeding, but in usual doses, breastfeeding is considered compatible [11].

There is no contraindication for Ampicillin to be administered at any gestational age. The main adverse effects (<2%) of this antibiotic include headaches, vomiting, nausea and vulvovaginal infections in pregnant women [7]. As Penicillin G Benzatin and Ampicillin are present in milk, the infant should be monitored for gastrointestinal disorders, such as diarrhea and thrush [11].

Cephalosporins

Cephalosporins, classified as B by the FDA, has the same structure and mechanism of action as penicillins, that is, the inhibition of bacterial wall synthesis, conferring a bactericidal action [2, 3].

In clinical practice, these antibiotics are grouped into five "generations" based on their spectrum of activity against aerobic bacilli, optional gram-negative and gram-positive bacteria [12]. The indications for each generation are described in Table **1**.

Among the cephalosporins, first-generation, second generation, third-generation (except Ceftibuten, Cefdinir) and fourth generation are present in breast milk, but they can be used with caution, always monitoring the infant for gastrointestinal effects. Cefdinir and Ceftibuten were not detected in milk and can be used [14].

All drugs, except Cefditoren and Loracarbef, interact with the intravesical BCG vaccine, being considered risk X in interaction; that is, this combination should be avoided. They also interact with the BCG vaccine (immunization), being considered risk C, because the benefits are greater than the harm, that is, therapy must be monitored, but there is no contraindication [14].

Table 1. Generations and indications of cephalosporins

First-Generation	
Cephalexin	Cellulite (not purulent)/erysipelas; not complicated cystitis; impetigo or ecthyma; streptococcal pharyngitis (group A). In pregnant women, it is used for asymptomatic bacteriuria, women who will go through normal birth and are classified as high risk for endocarditis, and in obese women after cesarean section to prevent infection [12 - 15].
Cefazolin	Mild to moderate cholecystitis; endocarditis; mild to moderate complicated and community-acquired intra-abdominal infections; general moderate to severe infections; mild infection cause by gram-positive cocci; perioperative prophylaxis; pneumococcal pneumonia; infection of the prosthetic joint caused by staphylococcus; skin and soft tissues infections caused by MSSA, including pyomyositis; streptococcal infections of the skin; simple urinary tract infection [7, 12 - 15].
Cefadroxil Cephradine	Infections caused by *Streptococcus, Staphylococcus aureus* [7, 10, 12].
Second Generation	
Cefuroxime Cefprozila Cefmetazol Loracarbef	Infections caused by *Escherichia coli, Klebsiella, Proteus, Haemophilus influenzae, Moraxella catarrhalis*. This generation has weak activity against *S. aureus*, but a strong activity against *Bacteroides fragilis* and other species of Bacteroides. In pregnancy , Cefuroxime is one of the antimicrobials used for prophylaxis of infections just before cesarean delivery [12].
Third Generation	
Ceftriaxone	Mild to moderate cholecystitis; endocarditis; mild to moderate complicated and community-acquired intra-abdominal infections; general moderate to severe infections; bacterial meningitis; mild to moderately severe pelvic inflammatory disease; community-acquired pneumonia (in combination with other antibiotics); infection of prosthetic joints; perioperative prophylaxis; complicated urinary tract infection (including pyelonephritis) [7, 12 - 15]. In pregnant women, it is indicated for the treatment of gonococcal infections, Lyme disease and prophylaxis for endocarditis in high-risk women [16].As this drug binds strongly to proteins, its use should be avoided before delivery due to the possibility of kernicterus [8].
Cefotaxime	Severe acute bacterial rhinosinusitis that requires hospitalization; septic arthritis; brain abscess; caesarean delivery; mild to moderate complicated intra-abdominal infections, including liver abscess (in combination with metronidazole); gonorrhea, simple infection of the cervix, urethra or rectum; lyme disease (as an alternative to ceftriaxone); bacterial meningitis; community-acquired; sepsis [7, 12 - 15].
Cefdinir Cefditoren Ceftibuten Cefpodoxime Ceftizoxime	Infections caused by *Enterobacteriaceae, Pseudomonas aeruginosa, Serratia, Neisseria gonorrhoeae, S. aureus, Streptococcus pneumoniae* and *Streptococcus pyogenes* [8].

(Table 1) contd.....

First-Generation	
Cefoperazone Ceftazidime	Infections caused by *Pseudomonas aeruginosa* [8].
Fourth Generation	
Cefepime	Intra-abdominal infection, infection associated to health care or high risk community-acquired; neutropenic fever in patients with high-risk cancer (absolute neutrophil count is expected to be ≤100 cells/mm3 for> 7 days, clinically unstable, or significant comorbidity) (empirical therapy); community-acquired pneumonia; hospital-acquired pneumonia or pneumonia associated with mechanical ventilation; moderate to severe skin and soft tissue infections; complicated acute urinary tract infection (including pyelonephritis) [12, 13, 15, 16].

In general, cephalosporins exhibit few adverse reactions in pregnant women, including hypersensitivity reactions, diarrhea, alcohol intolerance (those containing the methyl tetrazole group), significant renal toxicity (rare), severe hepatitis (rare). Since they are present in breast milk, infants should be monitored for gastrointestinal changes such as diarrhea and candidiasis [12].

Imipenem

This drug is part of the class of Carbapenems and is classified as C by the FDA [3]. This drug is considered bactericidal due to its action, which consists of interrupting the bacterial cell wall synthesis. Its spectrum covers a wide variety of anaerobes and aerobes, such as streptococci (except *S. pneumoniae* resistant to penicillin), enterococci (except *E. faecium* and non-beta-lactamase-producing strains), staphylococci and Listeria sensitive. Imipenem is indicated for urinary and gynecological infections, intra-abdominal infections, skin, soft tissue, bone and joint infections [17].

Regarding to pharmacological aspects, this drug is administered intravenously together with Cilastatin, a dehydropeptidase inhibitor, which prevents the renal metabolism of Imipenem. Its elimination is done by the kidneys and therefore its use in nephropathic patients should be monitored. It crosses the placenta and is present in milk, which is why the doctor must consider the risks of exposure to the fetus, the benefits of breastfeeding for the fetus and treatment for the mother [17, 18].

Adverse effects mainly include nausea and vomiting, but there may also be seizures in cases of patients with central nervous system injury and kidney failure receiving high doses. In addition, there may be a reduction in hematocrit, thrombocythemia and, in neonates, a reduction in hemoglobin, eosinophilia [17, 18].

Vancomycin

This drug is in the Glycopeptide class and is classified as C by the FDA. Its action consists of inhibiting the cell wall synthesis and it is generally bactericidal against sensitive strains except enterococci [2, 3, 17].

Its activity is effective against Gram-positive, being its main use in the treatment of methicillin-resistant *Staphylococcus aureus* (MRSA) organisms and severe staph infections in patients allergic to penicillin and cephalosporins [2]. In pregnant and breastfeeding women, it is used to treat *Clostridium difficile*, as well as in the prophylactic regimen in pregnant women who have MRSA [19].

As for pharmacological aspects, this drug is poorly absorbed orally, being generally administered intravenously. Its excretion occurs through the kidneys [17]. This drug crosses the placenta and fetal serum, amniotic fluid and cord blood. In pregnant women there may be an increase in the volume of distribution and an increase in plasma clearance, requiring higher doses to be effective [19]. Regarding use during breastfeeding, it is recommended only when the vancomycin relative infant dose (RID) is <10% [19].

Adverse effects include fever, rashes and phlebitis at the site of infection and hypersensitivity reactions [2]. The effects associated with ototoxicity and nephrotoxicity were not reported in the second and third semesters. In neonates gastrointestinal symptoms should be monitored [19].

Tetracyclines

This class is represented by Doxycycline, Minocycline, Tetracycline, Tigecycline. Its action consists of inhibiting the protein synthesis through its connection with the ribosomal subunit 30S and 50S, leading to the bacteriostatic effect. These drugs are effective against Gram-positive and Gram-negative, but they also act against *Rickettsia spp, Borrelia spp, Coxiella burnetii, Treponema spp, Chlamydia spp, Mycoplasma pneumoniae, Plasmodium spp, Vibrio cholerae, Vibrio vulnificus, Brucella spp, Calymmatobacterium granulomatis, Leptospira, Borrelia burgdorferi, Borrelia recurrentis, Burkholderia pseudomallei, Mycobacterium marinum, Entamoeba histolytica, Ehrlichia spp*, and *Anaplasma spp* [20].

This class is used as first-line therapy against rickettsiae, mycoplasmas and chlamydiae, and can also be used in skin and uncomplicated soft tissue infections [17].

Due to the high risk of hepatotoxicity in pregnant women and its accumulation in the teeth and bones of the fetus, almost all tetracyclines are contraindicated and, therefore, if this class is really necessary, as it is in Macular Fever, the drug of choice is Doxycycline, which has not been associated with teratogenic effects [20].

Tetracycline, doxycycline and minocycline in particular maintain excellent levels of activity against staphylococci, including MRSA [17].

Doxycycline is better than other drugs in this class because it can be administered orally or intravenously and is the only one that can be used in patients under eight years because other classes have been associated with risks of delayed bone growth [20].

Its greatest absorption is oral and its excretion is mainly renal [17]. This class has a good distribution in tissues and body fluids, being minocycline the most fat-soluble and tetracycline the least. All drugs cross the placenta and accumulate in the fetus' bone and teeth. In addition, they are released in large concentrations in milk, but their concentration in infants is very low due to the presence of calcium in breast milk [20, 21].

Adverse effects include gastrointestinal symptoms (abdominal discomfort, nausea, vomiting, anorexia and epigastric pain) mainly with intravenous administration of Tigecycline. Hepatotoxicity, a side effect of Tetracycline, Minocycline and Doxycycline, is rare, but it can be fatal [20], pregnant women are more prone to this complication [20, 21]. In pregnant and breastfeeding women, the use of this class can result in accumulation in the fetus' bone and teeth and permanently stain the infant's teeth [21]. In addition, it is contraindicated in terminal renal patients [20].

Chloramphenicol

Chloramphenicol is classified as class C by the FDA and has its systemic use reserved for more serious infections (*Haemophilus influenzae* resistant to other drugs, meningitis when penicillin is contraindicated and typhoid fever) and topical use in bacterial conjunctivitis [2]. This drug has a broad spectrum of action and is active against Gram-negative, Gram-positive and rickettsiae [22]. Its action consists of inhibiting the bacterial protein synthesis as it binds to the 50S subunit of the ribosome. This drug is considered bacteriostatic, although it can be bactericidal against *H. influenzae*, *Neisseria meningitidis* and *S. pneumoniae* [17].

This class has good distribution and oral or systemic absorption, and is excreted by the kidneys and inactivated by the liver [2]. This drug crosses the placenta and reaches concentrations similar to the mother's in the umbilical cord. The use in pregnant women during the third trimester should be monitored. Due to its great risks in newborns, this drug should not be used in breastfeeding women as it is present in breast milk [22]. The main side effect is spinal cord disease, causing idiosyncratic spinal depression and aplastic anemia, which results in pancytopenia when the drug is used in high doses or for prolonged periods, which can be fatal if treatment is not stopped [17, 23].

Chloramphenicol can decrease vitamin K synthesis, which could cause bleeding when used for a long time. In newborns it should be used with great care, because if not excreted/inactivated correctly, it can result in the gray syndrome, characterized by vomiting, diarrhea, flaccidity, low temperature and gray color. This syndrome has a high mortality rate [2], therefore all neonates should be monitored for gastrointestinal disorders, hemolysis and jaundice if this drug is really needed [22].

Aminoglycosides

The class of aminoglycosides is represented mainly by gentamicin, streptomycin, amikacin, tobramycin and neomycin and is used mostly against gram-negative enteric microorganisms and septicemia [2]. This class is effective against Gram-negative (*Enterobacteriaceae*, *Pseudomonas*, *Acinetobacter* *spp.* and *Haemophilus influenzae*), some Gram-positive (*Staphylococcus aureus)* and Mycobacteria (*Mycobacterium tuberculosis*, *Mycobacterium fortuitum*, *Mycobacterium abscessus* and *Mycobacterium chelonae*). Its action consists of inhibiting the bacterial protein synthesis, which results in a bactericidal effect. Beyond that, this class has a post-antibiotic effect, characterized by the permanence of bactericidal activity even after the serum concentration of the minimum inhibitory concentration drops [17]. Of all representatives of the class, amikacin has the largest spectrum, covering agents that are resistant to gentamicin and tobramycin and the most used is gentamicin [2, 17].

Regarding its distribution, it is reduced in pregnancy and, therefore, the use of doses over an extended interval is not recommended [24]. These are drugs that cross the placenta, but do not cross the blood-brain barrier. Its elimination is through the kidneys and the toxic effects are dose-dependent and therefore this class should be used with caution in nephropathic patients. Due to its poor oral absorption, there are no documented problems during breastfeeding despite being excreted in milk [17].

The adverse dose-dependent effects include mainly ototoxicity and nephrotoxicity. Otorhinolaryngological symptoms are vertigo, ataxia, loss of balance and hearing disorders and can be irreversible when used for a long time or in high doses. Nephrological effects, on the other hand, consist of elevated plasma creatinine, proteinuria and can even lead to dialysis, but in general are reversible [2, 17]. There is also a neuromuscular block, which is a rare condition and has been observed in association with anesthetics or other neuromuscular blockers. Streptomycin and tobramycin when administered to pregnant women in the third trimester can cause hearing loss in the newborn [17].

During pregnancy, Amikacin is the most suitable choice in case of need for aminoglycosides in a patient with multidrug-resistant tuberculosis and in multi antibiotic therapy against *Mycobacterium avium* in patients with cystic fibrosis [25]. They can also be used in the intrapartum period and infection intra-amniotic (Amikacin and Gentamicin) [24, 26].

Although the spectrum covers Gram-negative, it is not indicated for pregnant women in the treatment of simple urinary tract infection. However, the FDA classifies this drug as D, since it can result in its accumulation in fetal plasma and amniotic fluid when administered in the third trimester and associated side effects. Therefore this class should be used only in the absence of alternative therapies [3, 17].

Macrolide

Macrolides can have both bactericidal or bacteriostatic action, depending on the concentration, phase and type of microorganism. These antibiotics bind to the 50S subunit of bacterial ribosomes, leading to inhibition of bacterial protein synthesis [27]. Erythromycin is the macrolide with the greatest exposure for pregnant women. Among the newer macrolides, azithromycin shows greater effectiveness during pregnancy compared to clarithromycin or telithromycin [27, 28].

Erythromycin is a FDA category B drug. It is considered the antibiotic of choice for the treatment of PROM (<34 - 0/7 weeks of gestation), venereal lymphogranuloma in pregnancy, and long-term treatment or suppression of Bartonella infection in HIV-infected pregnant women. In addition, it is one of the antibiotics that can be used for the treatment of chancroid or inguinal granuloma and as an alternative agent for the treatment of chlamydia infections in pregnant women [28, 29].

Azithromycin is the same category as erythromycin. When used in pregnant women, it is indicated for the treatment of chronic obstructive pulmonary diseases; mycobacterial infection (non-tuberculous); pneumonia, acquired in the community; sexually transmitted infections (cervicitis, empirical therapy; chancroid; cervical infection with chlamydia trachomatis, urethra; gonococcal infection, without complications; urethritis, empirical therapy); and streptococcal pharyngitis (group A) (an alternative agent for patients allergic to severe penicillin) [27, 30].

Clarithromycin (FDA category C) is slightly more potent than erythromycin against strains susceptible to streptococci and staphylococci and has modest activity against *H. influenzae* and *N. gonorrhoeae*. This drug is quickly absorbed by the gastrointestinal tract (GIT) after oral administration, however, its first metabolization decreases its bioavailability to 50 to 55%. Metabolism is saturable, resulting in non-linear pharmacokinetics and longer half-lives after higher doses are administered [2, 3, 17].

The safety of use during pregnancy and breastfeeding has not yet been established, however, it is known that clarithromycin is excreted in breast milk; therefore, this product should not be used by pregnant or breastfeeding women, except in special cases [2].

Erythromycin, azithromycin and clarithromycin are associated with QT prolongation with ventricular tachycardia, among others, in particular Erythromycin, which presents these complications in the first trimester of pregnancy [31]. Among these agents, azithromycin is generally better tolerated followed by erythromycin [27, 17].

In addition, the Macrolides class is associated with the development of Infantile Hypertrophic Pyloric Stenosis in infants, especially in the first two weeks, and gastrointestinal tract effects such as loss of appetite, diarrhea, rash and drowsiness when exposed to macrolides through breast milk [14].

Sulphonamides

Sulfonamides are competitive inhibitors of hydropathioate synthase, the bacterial enzyme responsible for the incorporation of para-aminobenzoic acid (PABA) in dihydropteroic acid, the immediate precursor of folic acid. Trimethoprim produces a synergistic effect when used with a sulfonamide, as it repeatedly blocks the synthesis of tetrahydrofolate microorganisms [32].

The use of trimethoprim-sulfamethoxazole (category D) is avoided in the first trimester of pregnancy and in the short term, since this drug is an antagonist of folic acid, increasing the risk of neural tube defects. However, if the risk to the fetus is less than the benefit to the mother (for example, an HIV-infected pregnant woman needing prophylaxis/treatment for pneumocystis pneumonia), this drug should be used with supplemental folic acid [32].

Trimethoprim-sulfamethoxazole is indicated for the treatment of infections caused by gram-positive and gram-negative aerobic bacteria, *P. jirovecii*, in addition to *Burkholderia cepacia* (formerly *Pseudomonas cepacia*), *Stenotrophomonas maltophilia* (formerly *Xanthomonas maltophilia*), *Serratia marcescens*, *Nocardia spp.* and certain protozoa [32].

The most common adverse reactions to trimethoprim-sulfamethoxazole are related to the gastrointestinal tract (nausea, vomiting) and skin (rash and itching); decreased tubular creatinine secretion; renal tubular acidosis; hepatitis; hypoglycemia; hyponatremia and hemolysis in patients with glucose-6-phosphate dehydrogenase deficiency [32]. In infants, cases of kernicterus have been documented, since sulfonamide is present in milk, so it is recommended that both the doctor and the pregnant woman decide on either continuing therapy and suspending breastfeeding or the other way around [33].

Quinolones

There are several ways of dividing this class, but the most used classification is in generations, based on the antibacterial potential against pneumococcus and anaerobic organisms, so that the last generation is the most potent against these two groups [34]. Thus, the first generation is represented by Nalixylic Acid, Cinoxacin, the second is represented by Norfloxacino, Ciprofloxacino (the most potent against *Pseudomonas aeruginosa*), Lomefloxacino, Ofloxacino, Levofloxacino; third class is represented by Sparfloxacin, Gatifloxacino, Grepafloxacino; and fourth generation is represented by Trovafloxacin, Moxifloxacin and Gemifloxacin [34].

It is important to remember that the first generation did not have a fluorine molecule and with its addition from the second generation onwards, the quinolones can also be called fluoroquinolones [34].

This group is considered bactericidal and its action consists of inhibiting the bacterial topoisomerase II enzyme (DNA gyrase) and topoisomerase IV, both responsible for the transcription or replication of the organism [17, 35].

It is important to know that this class is being increasingly associated with resistance, which may be due to mutations in chromosomal genes or plasmids. Therefore, the use of fluoroquinolones should be limited in the following cases: urinary tract infection, typhoid and paratyphoid fever and infection by *Neisseria gonorrhoeae, Pseudomonas aeruginosa, Shigella spp* and *Campylobacter spp* [36].

In general, including in pregnant women, the adverse effects of this class are mainly associated with the gastrointestinal tract (nausea, vomiting, diarrhea and abdominal discomfort) and an increased risk of infection with *Clostridium difficile* due to its wide spectrum. Changes in the central nervous system (headache, dizziness, mood swings, insomnia, delirium, disorientation and attention disorders). Finally, regarding the cardiological system, there can be a QT prolongation resulting in Torsades de Pointes [36].

According to the FDA, this class is considered to be in C. There are studies done in animals that have documented changes in the development of cartilage and bones, but the very few studies done in pregnant women have not evidenced such change. However, studies carried out in pregnant women are limited to the moment of delivery, which does not confirm that these problems won't be developed in the newborn. For this reason, while there are no safe studies, it is recommended not to use it except in cases where this class is the only option [36].

Regarding breastfeeding, there are divergences in the literature as to whether this class can be used or not. As most antimicrobials in this class are present in breast milk and there may be a reduction in calcium absorption, we recommend deciding between continuing breastfeeding or medication, in order to avoid complications [37, 38].

Lincosamides

Among the antibiotics that belong to this class, clindamycin (category B) is an antibiotic that has been approved by the FDA for the treatment of anaerobic, streptococcal and staphylococcal infections in pregnant women [39]. The action of this drug consists of binding to the 50S subunit of the ribosomes of bacteria. Thus, it disrupts protein synthesis by interfering with the transpeptidation reaction, which inhibits early chain elongation [39].

Although it has been approved by the FDA, clindamycin has some restrictions on its use. In a study of pregnant women with bacterial vaginosis at 15.6 weeks of gestational age, the use of clindamycin (300 mg orally, twice daily for five days) was associated with a lower rate of miscarriages or premature births when compared to placebo. In contrast, the intravaginal clindamycin has been associated with an increased risk of premature birth, therefore, intravaginal clindamycin cream should be avoided in pregnant women [39].

As for treatment indications in pregnant women, clindamycin can be used for: osteomyelitis; pelvic inflammatory disease, severe septic arthritis due to *Staphylococcus aureus* (including MRSA) (alternative agent); skin and soft tissue infections; streptococcus (group A); and toxic shock syndrome (empirical therapy) [30, 40 - 43].

In general, including pregnant women, side effects do not have a defined frequency, but there may be hypotension, thrombophlebitis, metallic taste in the mouth, dermatological and gastrointestinal changes, among others. As this medication is present in milk, the infant should be monitored for gastrointestinal changes and blood stools. We strongly recommend that it is avoided during breastfeeding [44].

Rifampicin

This drug is of the antituberculous class, being classified by the FDA as C. Its action consists of binding and inhibiting the prokaryotic cells' DNA-dependent RNA polymerase, but not in eukaryotic [2]. The spectrum of Rifampicin covers *Mycobacterium tuberculosis*, *Mycobacterium leprae*, Gram-positive (*S. aureus*, coagulase negative staphylococci, *S. pyogenes*, *S. pneumoniae*, *viridans streptococci* and *Listeria monocytogenes*) and Gram-negative (*Legionella spp*, *Brucella spp*, *H. influenzae*, *Haemophilus ducreyi*, *Neisseria gonorrhoeae* and *N. meningitidis*).

In pregnant patients with tuberculosis, this drug is indicated when there is a moderate to high risk of infection of the fetus. They can also be used to treat Human Granulocytic Anaplasmosis (HGA) during pregnancy [45].

This medication has good oral absorption, which may be reduced or slowed in diabetic patients or those with HIV infection. It is well distributed in tissues and body fluids, including cerebrospinal fluid [45]. Its elimination is done through urine and bile [2]. This medicine crosses the placenta and milk and, therefore, if treatment with this drug is necessary, breastfeeding should be stopped. It is important to note that the dose of Rifampicin in milk is not sufficient to treat tuberculosis in the newborn [46].

Adverse effects include orange fluids, skin rashes, fever and gastrointestinal disorders (nausea, vomiting, diarrhea), mainly due to liver disease (jaundice, abnormal liver function, increased degradation of warfarin, glucocorticoids, narcotic analgesics, antidiabetics oral drugs, dapsone and estrogens) [2, 45]. When administered in the third trimester, they can cause postpartum hemorrhage in neonates and mothers [46].

Others

Metronidazole

Metronidazole is a derivative of nitroimidazole with activity against a wide variety of anaerobic organisms, including protozoa, parasites and bacteria. It is clinically effective in trichomoniasis, amoebiasis and giardiasis; as well as in a variety of infections caused by mandatory anaerobic bacteria, such as *Clostridium*, Bacteroides; facultative anaerobic bacteria, such as *Helicobacter pylori* and *Gardnerella vaginalis* [47].

When used against mandatory anaerobes, its mechanism consists of a four-step process, which includes entry into the body, reducing activation by intracellular transport proteins, interactions with intracellular targets and rupture of cytotoxic intermediates [47].

Metronidazole has been approved and classified by the FDA as a category B drug. However, its use in pregnancy is somewhat controversial. As there are currently no adequate studies to demonstrate safety in pregnant women and there are reports of lip leporin in neonates and carcinogenesis in animal species, metronidazole should only be used during pregnancy if clearly necessary and should be avoided during the first trimester of pregnancy [35, 47, 48].

In general, including in pregnant women, the side effects most commonly associated with systemic metronidazole therapy are gastrointestinal (such as nausea, anorexia, vomiting, diarrhea, abdominal cramps, constipation), neurological (such as peripheral neuropathy, confusion, dizziness) and immunologic (hypersensitive reactions) [47]. As it is present in milk, breastfeeding must be suspended during its use and up to three days afterwards, since it is associated with oral and perianal candidiasis, diarrhea in infants [47, 48].

Nitrofurantoin

Nitrofurantoin is a synthetic nitrofuran used mainly in prophylaxis (for recurrent infections) and in the treatment of urinary tract infections in pregnant women, and is considered a category B by the FDA. It is activated through enzymatic reduction and is responsible for causing damage to bacterial DNA, especially strains of *Escherichia coli* and *enterococci* [49].

The use of nitrofurantoin during the first trimester of pregnancy should be limited to situations in which there are no alternative therapies and, preferably, for the shortest effective time for confirmed infections. This drug is contraindicated in pregnant women at term (38 to 42 weeks of gestation), during labor, or when its onset is imminent due to the possibility of hemolytic anemia of the newborn. In addition, the use of Nitrofurantoin in pregnant women up to 30 days previous to delivery is associated with neonatal jaundice [50]. Its use should also be avoided in pregnant patients with G6PD deficiency and, instead, there should be the option of alternative antibiotics [49].

In general, including pregnant women, the most common adverse events consist of nausea, vomiting, diarrhea and hypersensitive reactions (chills, fever, leuko- penia, granulocytopenia, hemolytic anemia (associated with G6PD deficiency), cholestatic jaundice and hepatocellular damage) [49]. Breastfeeding women using Nitrofurantoin should either choose to discontinue breastfeeding or the drug, since the infant may develop hemolytic anemia, in addition to gastrointestinal effects such as diarrhea and oral candidiasis [50].

Phosphomycin

Fosfomycin (category B) is a derivative of phosphonic acid and is considered bactericidal because it inhibits the synthesis of the bacterial wall through inactivation of the enzyme pyruvyl transferase [51].

The choice of the antimicrobial agent must take into account safety during pregnancy, especially during the specific phase of the pregnancy. In several studies, fosfomycin has been shown to be safe during pregnancy. When administered as a single dose, it was well tolerated and no adverse fetal effects were observed [15].

Among the indications for this antimicrobial, we emphasize the treatment of asymptomatic bacteriuria and simple acute cystitis. However, although fosfomycin is included in clinical practice guidelines as a first-line agent for simple acute cystitis, reduced efficacy has been reported when compared to other first-line agents [15, 51].

The general side effects of this class, including in pregnant women, include headache, dizziness, diarrhea, nausea, vomiting, vaginitis, dysmenorrhea, among others. In infants, gastrointestinal changes such as candidiasis and diarrhea should be monitored [52].

ANTIFUNGALS

The antifungal agents available cause effects on the synthesis of cell wall and membrane components, on the permeability of the membrane, on the synthesis of nucleic acids and on the function of the microtubic/mitotic spindle [53].

They can be divided into five classes: polyethylene, azole, allylamine, echinocandins and others. During pregnancy, some classes will be restricted to use in the first trimester or in reduced doses or restriction of use throughout pregnancy. It is important to be aware of the proper use of each drug to avoid its teratogenic effect in pregnancy, if it exists [53]. Table **2** lists the classification of antifungals according to their mechanisms of action.

Table 2. Classification of antifungals.

Antifungals that Interfere in the Cell Membrane			
Polyene	**Amphotericin B (Category B of FDA)** **Nystatin (Category C of FDA)**		
Azole (Category C of FDA)	Systems Fluconazole Itraconazole Voriconazole Posaconazole Isavuconazole	Topics	
		Clotrimazole Econazole Miconazole Terconazole Butoconazole	Tioconazole ketoconazole Oxiconazole Sulconazole Sertaconazole
Allylamine	Terbinafine (Category B of FDA)		
Morpholine Derivatives	Amorolfina (Category C of FDA)		
Antifungals that Interfere in The The Cell Wall			
Echinocandins **(Category C of FDA)**	Caspofungina Micafungina Anidulafungina		
Polyoxins and Nicomicins **(Category C of FDA)**			
Antifungal Agents that Interfere in The Mitosis			
Griseofulvin **(Equivalent to category D of FDA)**			
Antifungals that Interfere in the Synthesis of Nucleic Acid			
Flucitosina			
Antifungal Agents that Interfere in The Protein Synthesis			
Sordarinas			
Ciclopirox Olamine (Category B of FDA)			

Each member of the azole class exhibits a unique spectrum of activity, although fluconazole, itraconazole, voriconazole, posaconazole and isavuconazole show similar activity against most Candida species [53].

Oral azole therapy is especially avoided during the first trimester because, although studies are still unclear, there is a risk of miscarriage; and high doses seem to increase the risk of birth defects. Because it is an effective alternative to oral dosing, topical therapy is preferable in vaginal treatment until further studies are available to support the safety of low-dose oral treatment [54].

In the case of Fluconazole, there are some literary divergences regarding its use in pregnancy. For some authors, the oral use of fluconazole for vaginal candidiasis is not recommended in pregnant women at any gestational age [55].

Other studies report that after exposure during the first trimester, malformations were observed in fetuses (including brachycephaly, abnormal face, abnormal development of the cap, cleft palate, femoral curvature, thin ribs and long bones, arthrogryposis and congenital heart disease) when fluconazole was used in higher doses ($\geq$ 400 mg/day) for long periods of time [54, 56].

In addition, a cohort study of more than 3,300 women receiving low-dose oral fluconazole (150-300 mg) in the first and second trimesters reported an approximately 50% increase in the risk of miscarriage in exposed women compared to unexposed women or women treated with vaginal azole. Regarding birth defects, no increase has been reported in women treated with a single low dose of fluconazole 150 mg [54].

In the polyethylene class, amphotericin B is considered as a category B by the FDA, together with terbinafine (representative of allylamines). However, amphotericin B is restricted to the treatment of severe systemic fungal diseases in pregnant women, as it crosses the placenta and enters the fetal circulation. Terbinafine, which is indicated for the treatment of onychomycosis, can be used after pregnancy [56, 57].

Oral nystatin (representative of the polyethylene class) and the echinocandin class are classified by the FDA as category C, the risk to the fetus cannot be ruled out. As there are no adequate studies of these drugs in pregnant women, they should only be used if the potential benefit justifies the risk to the fetus. However, the use of vaginal nystatin during pregnancy has not reported adverse events in the fetus or newborn [29, 58].

ANTIVIRAL AGENTS

Viruses are mandatory unicellular and intracellular microorganisms that consist of DNA or RNA and a protein envelope. Some viruses may still have a lipid structure that provides greater protection of the genetic material. Antiviral agents were created to act on specific virus replication events or on the production of proteins and genetic material necessary for the survival of that parasite, and not of the human host cell [59].

Herpesviridae

In this group, we have Acyclovir, and the oldest Ganciclovir and Fanciclovir. These drugs are nucleoside analogs that selectively inhibit the replication of the herpes simplex virus types 1 and 2 (HSV-1, HSV-2) and the varicella-zoster virus (VZV). These drugs are classified as category B by the FDA and although there are no controlled studies, large observational studies can, as Danish researchers published in 2010, claim that antiviral therapy was not associated with an increased risk of birth defect [60].

Therefore, animal and human data on exposure to acyclovir during pregnancy, including the first trimester, suggest that this medication is safe at all stages of pregnancy. The data are more limited, although comforting about the use of valacyclovir. There is minimal human data on exposure to famciclovir during pregnancy [61, 62].

Antiretrovirals

HIV drugs should be used on all HIV-infected individuals, including pregnant women, regardless of lymphocyte count or viral load. However, in pregnant women, there are additional precautions to prevent vertical transmission [63, 64].

As we know, there are now countless drugs of different classes to combat HIV replication. In the class of non-nucleoside reverse transcriptase inhibitors, we have Efavirenz, which is part of the therapeutic regimen recommended by the World Health Organization (WHO) and is safe for use in pregnant women. There are also inhibitors of nucleoside reverse transcriptase, represented by Abacavir, Emtricitabine, Lamivudine, Tenofovir (FDA Category C) and Zidovudine. As for the protease inhibitors, we have safe representatives in pregnancy Atazanavir, Darunavir, Lopinavir-ritonavir. Finally, the class of integrin inhibitors consists of Raltegravir and Dolutegravir, which are used preferentially in the second and third trimesters of pregnancy [63, 65].

Briefly, in general, the known benefits outweigh the potential risks to the fetus. However, the decision on therapy must be specific to the pregnant woman and must take into account the pharmacokinetic changes and possible toxicity for the mother and the fetus [64, 66].

Anti-influenza

As influenza infection is associated with an increased risk of adverse events in the fetus and mother, prophylaxis and treatment of this disease in pregnant women is important.

Currently, the best cost-effective option is the influenza A vaccine, but there are also antivirals that can be used. Rimantadine and Amantadine are effective when acting against influenza A, but are associated with teratogenic effects in animals and are therefore considered class C. Amantadine is present in the breast milk and associated with reduced prolactin production. and that is why it should be avoided [67, 68]. Rimantadine is not excreted in milk but it is also not recommended [67, 69].

There are also two other classes of extreme importance in influenza infection during pregnancy. Oseltamivir and Zanamivir act by selectively inhibiting the neuraminidases of influenza A and B viruses. Both are used in the treatment and prevention of influenza A and B infection and are associated with a reduction in subsequent adult hospitalization, reduced disease duration, rapid functional recovery and reduced chances of complications [17].

As infection by influenza is associated with an increased risk of adverse events in fetus and mother, Olsetamivir is recommended for treatment and prophylaxis in pregnant women and up to 2 weeks postpartum [70] whereas Zanamivir can be used, but it is not the first line [71].

Zanamivir is associated with serious adverse respiratory effects, including death, in patients with previous respiratory diseases. The side effects of Zanamivir in patients without these diseases are mild and are mainly associated with the respiratory and gastrointestinal tracts. The effects of Olsetamivir mainly consist of nausea, abdominal discomfort, headache but they tend to disappear after 1-2 days of use [17].

ANTIMALARIAL AGENTS

Malaria is responsible for around 900,000 deaths each year worldwide. This disease is more serious in pregnant women since it increases the risk of miscarriage, premature birth, low birth weight, congenital infections and perinatal death [72]. It is an infection caused by single-celled parasitic protozoa of the genus *Plasmodium*. The species most related to the disease in humans are *P. falciparum* and *P. vivax*. There are currently three classes of antimalarial drugs: Artemisinins and derivatives, Atovaquone/Proguanil, and Primaquine [73, 74].

Its representatives are artemisinins, chloroquine, mefloquine, quinine/quinidine, pyrimethamine, sulfadoxine and tetracycline (FDA Category C). They are very potent and fast-acting drugs, inducing the best parasitic clearance and resolution of fever among all antimalarials [74]. Among this class, the drugs that cannot be used due to their risk in pregnant women are Antifolates, atovaquone-proguanil, artemer-lumefantrine and those with teratogenic risk to the fetus are tetracyclines, doxycycline, primaquine, mefloquine.

Most studies agree that drugs in this class have an activity that culminates in the formation of highly toxic adult heme parasites, in addition to generating radicals that alkylate and oxidize proteins and lipids in parasitized erythrocytes. Due to its fast and potent activity, this class of drugs is indicated for the treatment of severe *falciparum* malaria. However, they should not be used for chemoprophylaxis, given their very short half-life [75, 76].

During the first trimester of pregnancy, in the presence of malaria infection (which type), the only drug of choice in this class is quinine, which is associated with clindamycin. During the last two trimesters, all drugs in this class can be used [74].

Regarding side effects, we should pay attention to Quinins, since they can cause hypoglycemia in pregnant women, leading to nausea, vomiting, and dizziness. In addition, there is still a rare triad of disorders of the hematological system, consisting of hemolysis, hemoglobinemia and hemoglobinuria. Infants should be monitored for jaundice and hemolysis, especially if they are <1 month [72].

ANTHELMINTIC AGENTS

Pathogenic worms for humans are metazoan and can be classified into nematodes and two types of flatworms (trematodes and cestodes) [77].

Anthelmintics are drugs used not only to treat a symptomatic infection, but also as prophylaxis in endemic regions. However, in pregnant women, it is recommended to leave the treatment after delivery, since its use may be associated with changes in the fetus that have not been specified [78].

Ivermectin

This drug is classified as C by FDA and is a derivative of the class of avermectins, which results from the fermentation by Streptomyces avermitilis [79]. Its mechanism of action is related to the opening of chloride channels sensitive to glutamate present in the helminth. It is the drug of choice for the treatment of onchocerciasis and strongyloidiasis, but it is also effective in the treatment of ascariasis and trichuriasis [59].

This medication should not be used in pregnant women since there are few studies about its safety, in addition to being associated with the appearance of eczema in neonates [78]. In breastfeeding women, there are differences in the literature, but we recommend that it should not be used [79, 80].

Benzimidazole (BZs)

This class includes thiabendazole (FDA Category C), mebendazole, and albendazole. The mechanism of action is related to the inhibition of microtubule polymerization by binding to B-tubulin.

Albendazole and mebendazole (FDA Category C) have excellent activity against neurocysticercosis, echinococcosis, ascariasis, hookworms and trichuriasis. They can also be used in ectoparasites, such as the infection of migrating larvae [79]. Thiabendazole also has a wide spectrum, but its use is limited due to the frequent side effects associated with nausea, vomiting, itching, headache, dizziness, hepatitis and hypersensitivity reactions [79].

This class should be avoided in pregnant women when possible. However, when necessary, albendazole and mebendazole should be the drugs of choice and can be used in the second and third trimesters of pregnancy [79].

Praziquantel (FDA Category B)

This medication is mainly active in schistosomiasis, as it causes helminth paralysis and consequently its death [59]. It should only be used in pregnant women who are in the second or third trimester of pregnancy. Its side effects are uncommon and include nausea, vomiting, itching, headache and dizziness [79].

CONCLUSION

The treatment of infections caused by bacteria, fungi, viruses and other microorganisms is important, as it can prevent complications such as prematurity, vertical transmission and maternal or fetal death. However, not all infectious agents are safely assessed for serious adverse effects for pregnant women and fetuses. Therefore, knowledge of the classification of these agents and the potential risks and benefits of use during pregnancy is essential to avoid the adverse effects that bring serious problems to the mother-fetus binomial.

CONSENT FOR PUBLICATION

Not applicable.

CONFLICT OF INTEREST

The authors declare no conflict of interest, financial or otherwise.

ACKNOWLEDGEMENTS

Declared none.

REFERENCES

[1]   Content and format of labeling for human prescription drug and biological products; Requirements for pregnancy and lactation labeling. Final rule. Fed Regist 2014; 79(233): 72063-103.

[2]   Rang HP, Ritter JM, Flower RJ, *et al.* Rang & dale pharmacology: Drugs used to treat infection and cancer. 8th ed. Rio de Janeiro: Elsevier 2016; pp. 630-639, 656, 658-666, 674.

[3]   Content and Format of Labeling for Human Prescription Drug and Biological Products; Requirements for Pregnancy and Lactation Labeling. USA: US Food and Drugs administration; 2014 May 12. Overview of the Final Rule, Including Significant Changes to the Proposed Rule 2014. https://www.federalregister.gov/d/2014-28241/p-90

[4]   Letourneau AR. Penicillin, antistaphylococcal penicillins, and broad-spectrum penicillins. David C Hooper 2019. https://www.uptodate.com/contents/penicillin-antistaphylococcal-penicillins-and-b-oad-spectrum-penicillins

[5]   Letourneau AR. Beta-lactam antibiotics: Mechanisms of action and resistance and adverse effects. David C Hooper; [revised 1st Sep 2020 2019. Available from: https://www.uptodate.com/contents/beta-lactam-antibiotics-mechanisms-of-action-and-resistance -and-adverse-effects

[6]   Norwitz ER, Hicks CB. Syphilis in pregnancy. Charles J Lockwood 2019. Available from: https://www.uptodate.com/contents/syphilis-in-pregnancy

[7]   Lipsky B, Berendt A, Cornia P, *et al.* Infectious diseases society of america (ISDA) clinical practice guideline for the diagnosis and treatment of diabetic. Clin Infect Dis 2012; 55(10): e1279-82. https://pubmed.ncbi.nlm.nih.gov/23091044/

[8]   Lexicomp.Penicillin G (intravenous and short-acting intramuscular): Drug information. Lexicomp 2020. Available from: https://www.uptodate.com/contents/penicillin-g-intravenous-and-short-acting-intramuscular-druginformation?=penicilinas&source=search_result& selectedTitle=10~150&usage_type=default&display_rank=5#F5720623%20-

[9]   Lexicomp. Amoxicillin: Drug information. Lexicomp 2020. Available from: https://www.uptodate. com/ contents/amoxicillin-drug-information? search=amoxicilina&source= panel_search_result &selectedTitle=1~148&usage_type=panel&kp_tab=drug_general&display_rank=1#F5720643

[10] Larson L, File TM. Treatment of respiratory infections in pregnant women. Vincenzo Berghella 2019. Available from: https://www.uptodate.com/contents/syphilis-in-pregnancy

[11] Lexicomp. Ampicillin: Drug information. Lexicomp 2020. Available from: https://www.uptodate.com/contents/ampicillin-drug-information?search=ampicilina%20drug&source=panel_search_result&selectedTitle=1~148&usage_type=panel&kp_tab=drug_general&display_rank=1#F134941

[12] Letourneau AR. Letourneau AR. Cephalosporins: Hopper DC 2020 . Available from: https://www.uptodate.com/contents/cephalosporins

[13] Stevens DL, Bisno AL, Chambers HF, *et al.* Infectious diseases society of America (IDSA). Practice guidelines for the diagnosis and management of skin and soft tissue infections. Clin Infect Dis 2014; 59(2): e10-52.
[http://dx.doi.org/10.1093/cid/ciu296] [PMID: 24973422]

[14] Drugs and Lactation Database (LactMed): Drugs and Lactation Database (LactMed): National Library of Medicine (USA): Bethesda; Drugs and Lactation Database 2016. Available from: https://www.ncbi.nlm.nih.gov/books/NBK501375/

[15] Hooton TM, Gupta K. Urinary tract infections and asymptomatic bacteriuria in pregnancy. SB Calderwood, Lockwood CJ 2019. Available from: https://www.uptodate.com/contents/dosing-and-administration-of-parenteral-aminoglycosides

[16] Lexicomp. Ceftriaxone: Drug information. Lexicomp 2020. Available from: https://www.uptodate.com/contents/ceftriaxone-drug-information?search=ceftriaxona&source=panel_search_result&selectedTitle=1~148&usage_type=panel&kp_tab=drug_general&display_rank=1

[17] Brunton LL, Chabner BA, Knollmann BC, *et al.* Goodman & Gilman's pharmacological basis of therapeutics: Chemotherapy of Microbial Diseases. 12th ed. New York: McGraw-Hill Medical 2012; pp. 1421-1427, 1470-1474, 1529, 1539-1542, 1545.

[18] Lexicomp. Imipenem and cilastatin: Drug information. Lexicomp 2020. Available from: https://www.uptodate.com/contents/imipenem-and-cilastatin-drug-information?search=cilastatina&source=search_result&selectedTitle=2~27&usage_type=default&display_rank=2#F182034

[19] Lexicomp.Vancomycin: Drug information. Lexicomp 2020. Available from: https://www.uptodate.com/contents/vancomycin-drug-information?search=antibi%C3%B3ticos%20glicopept%C3%ADdeos&source=search_result&selectedTitle=4~150&usage_type=default&display_rank=4#F6833811

[20] May DB. Tetracyclines. Hooper DC 2020. Available from: https://www.uptodate.com/contents/tetracyclines?search=tetraciclina&source=search_result&selectedTitle=2~148&usage_type=default&display_rank=3#H1

[21] Lexicomp.Tetracycline: Drug information . Lexicomp 2020. Available from: https://www.uptodate.com/contents/tetracycline-drug-information?search=tetraciclina&source=search_result&selectedTitle=1~148&usage_type=panel&kp_tab=drug_general&display_rank=1#F226280

[22] Lexicomp. Chloramphenicol: Drug information. Lexicomp 2020. Available from: https://www.uptodate.com/contents/chloramphenicol-drug-information?search=cloranfenicol&source=panel_search_result&selectedTitle=1~84&usage_type=panel&kp_tab=drug_general&display_rank=1

[23] Lexicomp. Chloramphenicol: Drug information. Lexicomp 2020. Available from: https://www.uptodate.com/contents/chloramphenicol-drug-information?search=cloranfenicol&source=panel_search_result&selectedTitle=1~84&usage_type=panel&kp_tab=drug_general&display_rank=1

[24] Drew RH. Dosing and administration of parenteral aminoglycosides: Chemotherapeutic drugs. Hooper DC 2020. Available from: https://www.uptodate.com/contents/dosing-and-administration-of-parenteral-aminoglycosides

[25] Lexicomp. Amikacin (systemic): Drug information. Lexicomp 2020. Available from:

https://www.uptodate.com/contents/amikacin-systemic-dr-
g-information?search=amicacina&source=panel_sea rch_result&selectedTitle=1~103&usage_type=pa
nel&display_rank=1#F51959356

[26]   Tita ATN, *et al.* Intraamniotic infection (clinical chorioamnionitis or triple I). Vincenzo Berghella
2020.   Available   from: https://www.uptodate.com/contents/intraamniotic-infection-clinic-
l-chorioamnionitis-or-triple-i

[27]   Graziani AL. Azithromycin and clarithromycin. Hooper DC (Ed.). 2020. Available from:
https://www.uptodate.com/contents/intraamniotic-infection-clinical-chorioamnionitis-or-triple-i

[28]   Committee on Adolescent Health Care, Committee on Gynecologic Practice, Expedited Partner
Therapy.   ACOG   Committee   Opinion   2018;   131(6):   190-3.   Available   from:
https://www.acog.org/en/Clinical/Clinical%20Guidance/Committee%20Opinion/Articles
/2018/06/Expedited%20Partner%20Therapy

[29]   Mofenson LM, Brady MT, Danner SP, *et al.* Guidelines for the prevention and treatment of
opportunistic infections among HIV-Exposed and HIV-Infected children: Recommendations from
CDC, the national institutes of health, the HIV medicine association of the infectious diseases society
of America, the pediatric infectious diseases society, and the American academy of pediatrics. Author
manuscript   2009;   58(11):   1.   Available   from:
https://www.ncbi.nlm.nih.gov/pmc/articles/PMC2821196/

[30]   Workowski KA, Bolan GA. Sexually transmitted diseases treatment guidelines. Morbidity and
Mortality   Weekly   Report   (MMWR)   2018.   Available   from:
https://www.ncbi.nlm.nih.gov/pmc/articles/PMC5885289/

[31]   Lexicomp. Erythromycin (systemic): Drug information. Lexicomp 2020. Available from:
https://www.uptodate.com/contents/erythromycin-systemic-drug-information?
search=eritromicin&source=panel_search_result&selectedTitle=1~142&usage_type=panel&display_r
ank=1

[32]   May DB, *et al.* Trimethoprim-sulfamethoxazole: An overview. Hooper DC 2018. Available from:
https://www.uptodate.com/contents/trimethoprim-sulfamethoxazole-an-overview

[33]   Montanaro A, N Franklin Adkinson JR, *et al.* Sulfonamide allergy in HIV-uninfected patients. 2020.
Available from: https://www.uptodate.com/contents/trimethoprim-sulfamethoxazole-an-overview

[34]   Andriole VT. Andriole VT. The Quinolones: Past, Present, and Future. Clinical Infectious Diseases.
2005; 41: 113-9. Available from: https://academic.oup.com/cid/article/41/Supplement_2/S113/307164
[http://dx.doi.org/10.1086/428051]

[35]   Katzung BG, Trevor AJ, *et al.* Basic & clinical pharmacology: Chemotherapeutic drugs . 13th ed. New
York: McGraw-Hill Medical 2017; pp. 865-1130. ISBN: 85-8055-597-4.

[36]   Hooper   DC.   Fluoroquinolones.   Stephen   B   Calderwood   2019.   Available   from:
https://www.uptodate.com/contents/fluoroquinolones?search
=quinolonas%20gera%C3%A7%C3%B5es&source=search_result&selectedTitle=1~150&usage_type
=default&display_rank=1#H4231855561

[37]   Drugs   and   Lactation   Database.   LacMed;   Norfloxacin   2018.   Available   from:
https://www.ncbi.nlm.nih.gov/books/NBK501054/

[38]   Lexicomp.   Norfloxacin   (United   States):   Drug   information.   2020.   Available   from:
https://www.uptodate.com/contents/norfloxacin-united-states-not-available-
drug-information?search=norflo xacino&usage_type=panel&kp_tab=drug_general&source=panel_sea
rch_result&select edTitle=1~28&display_rank=1

[39]   Pernia S, DeMaagd G. The new pregnancy and lactation labeling rule. Pharmacy and therapeutics.
2016; 41(11): 713-5. Available from: https://www.ncbi.nlm.nih.gov/pmc/articles/PMC5083079/#

[40]   Berbari EF, Kanj SS, Kowalski TJ, *et al.* 2015 Infectious Diseases Society of America (IDSA) Clinical
Practice Guidelines for the Diagnosis and Treatment of Native Vertebral Osteomyelitis in Adults. Clin

Infect Dis 2015; 61(6): e26-46.
[http://dx.doi.org/10.1093/cid/civ482] [PMID: 26229122]

[41]   Stevens DL. Invasive group A streptococcal infection and toxic shock syndrome: Treatment and prevention. Morven S Edwards; 2020. Available from: https://www.upto date.com/contents/invasive-group-a-streptococcal-infection-and-toxic-shock-syndr ome-treatment-and-prevention

[42]   Goldenberg DL, Sexton DJ. Goldenberg DL, Sexton DJ. Septic arthritis in adults. Sexton DJ 2020. Available from: https://www.uptodate.com/contents/septic-arthritis-in-adults

[43]   Stevens DL, Bisno AL, Chambers HF, *et al.* Practice guidelines for the diagnosis and management of skin and soft tissue infections. 2014 update by the Infectious Diseases Society of America. 2014; (59): 147-59. Available from: https://pubmed.ncbi.nlm.nih.gov/24973422/
[http://dx.doi.org/10.1093/cid/ciu444.]

[44]   Johnson M. Clindamycin: An overview. Hooper DC 2020. Available from: https://www.uptodate.com/contents/clindamycin-an-overview?search=https%20www% 20uptodate%20com%20contents%20clindamycin%20systemic%20drug%20information%20search%2 0clindamycin%20source%20panel%20search%20result%20selectedtitle%201%20145%20usage%20t ype%20panel%20display%20rank%201%20f8008064&source=search_result&selectedTitle=1~150&u sage_type=default&display_rank=1

[45]   Drew RH. Rifamycins (rifampin, rifabutin, rifapentine). Bernardo J 2020. Available from: https://www.uptodate.com/contents/rifamycins-rifampin-rifabutin-rifapentine/ contributors

[46]   Lexicomp. Rifampin (rifampicin): Drug information. 2020. Available from: https://www.uptodate.com/contents/rifamycins-rifampin-rifabutin-rifapentine/contributors

[47]   Johnson M. Metronidazole: An overview. 2019. Available from: https://www.uptodate.com/contents/metronidazole -an-overview

[48]   Lexicomp.Metronidazole (systemic): Drug information. 2020. Available from: https://www.uptodate.com/contents/amikacin-systemic-drug-information?search=amicacina& source=panel_search _result&selectedTitle=1~103&usage_type=panel&display_rank=1#F51959356

[49]   Stevens DL, Bisno AL, Chambers HF, *et al.* Infectious Diseases Society of America (IDSA). Practice guidelines for the diagnosis and management of skin and soft tissue infections. Clin Infect Dis 2014; 59(2): e10-52.
[http://dx.doi.org/10.1093/cid/ciu296] [PMID: 24973422]

[50]   Lexicomp. Nitrofurantoin: Drug information. 2020. Available from: https://www.uptodate.com/contents/nitrofurantoin-drug-information?search=nitrofuran to%C3%ADna &source=panel_search_result&selectedTitle=1~61&usage_type=panel&kp_tab=drug_general&displa y_rank=1#F201977

[51]   Angela H, Anna K, Adi T. Effect of 5-day nitrofurantoin *vs* single-dose fosfomycin on clinical resolution of uncomplicated lower urinary tract infection in women: A randomized clinical trial. JAMA. 2018; 17: 1781-9. Available from: https://jamanetwork.com/ journals/jama/fullarticle /2679131

[52]   Lexicomp. Fosfomycin: Drug information. 2020. Available from: https://www.uptodate.com/contents/fosfomycin-drug-information?search=fosfomicina&source =panel_search_result&selectedTitle=1~19&usage_type=panel&kp_tab=drug_general&display_ rank=1#F7277079

[53]   Pharmacology of azoles. Carol A Kauffman; Mechanism of action 2020. Available from: https://www.uptodate.com/contents/pharmacology-of-azoles

[54]   Robert L Barbieri, Carol A Kauffman, Carol A Kauffman. *Candida vulvovaginitis*: Treatment. Special populations: Breastfeeding women 2020. Available from: https://www.uptodate.com/contents/candida-vulvovaginitis-treatment

[55]   Centers for Disease Control and Prevention. 2015 Sexually Transmitted Diseases Treatment

Guidelines. Sexually Transmitted Diseases (STDs): Special populations. 2019; 60(13) Available from: https://www.cdc.gov/std/tg2015/specialpops.htm

[56] Pappas PG, Kauffman CA, Andes DR. Infectious Diseases Society of America (IDSA). Clinical Practice Guideline for the Management of Candidiasis: 2016 Update by the Clinical Infectious Diseases. 2016; 62(4): e1-e50. Available from: https://academic.oup.com/cid/article/62/4/e1/2462830

[57] Novartis Pharmaceuticals Canada Inc. LAMISIL: Product monograph. Canada: Novartis Pharmaceuticals Canada Inc 2019. Available from: https://www.novartis.ca/sites/www.novartis.ca/files/lamisil_scrip_e.pdf

[58] US Food and Drug Administration. Highlights of prescribing information: Mycamine. 2015. Available from: https://www.accessdata.fda.gov/drugsatfda_docs/label/2016/021506s019lbl.pdf

[59] Tavares W. Antibióticos e Quimioterápicos para o Clínico. 3rd rev. ed., Atheneu 2014. https://cardiologiamedicinaumsa.files.wordpress.com/2017/07/antibioticos-y-quimioterapicos-para-el-clinico.pdf

[60] Pasternak B. Use of acyclovir, valacyclovir, and famciclovir in the first trimester of pregnancy and the risk of birth defects. JAMA 2010; 304(8): 859-66. Available from: https://jamanetwork.com/journals/jama/fullarticle/186468#:~:text=Conclusion%20In %20this %20large%20nationwide,simplex%20and%20herpes%20zoster%20infections

[61] Acyclovir: An overview: Use in pregnancy. Hirsch MS 2020. Available from: https://www.uptodate.com/contents/acyclovir-an-overview

[62] Polso A, Lassiter J, Nagel J. Impact of hospital guideline for weight-based antimicrobial dosing in morbidly obese adults and comprehensive literature review. J Clin Pharm Ther 2014; 39(6): 584-608. Available from: https://pubmed.ncbi.nlm.nih.gov/25203631/

[63] Henry J. Guidelines for the use of antiretroviral agents in HIV-infected adults and adolescents, January 28, 2000 by the Panel on Clinical Practices for Treatment of HIV Infection. J Med Pract 2000; 5(2): 79-104. Available from: https://pubmed.ncbi.nlm.nih.gov/12322315/

[64] Lynne MM. Antiretroviral selection and management in pregnant women with HIV in resource-rich settings. Art selection and management: General principles 2020. Available from: https://www.uptodate.com/contents/antiretroviral-selection-and-management-in-pregnant-women - with-hiv-in-resource-rich-settings

[65] Li N, Sando MM, Spiegelman D, *et al.* Antiretroviral therapy in relation to birth outcomes among HIV-infected women: A cohort study. J Infect Dis 2015; 213(7): 64-1057. Available from: https://pubmed.ncbi.nlm.nih.gov/26265780/

[66] Lynne MM. Safety and dosing of antiretroviral medications in pregnancy. Integrase inhibitors: Fetal safety 2020. Available from: https://www.uptodate.com/contents/safety-and-dosing-of-antiretrov-ral-medications-in-pregnancy

[67] Ministério da Saúde. Amamentação e uso de drogas. Amamentação e uso de medicamentos e outras substâncias. 2017; (2): 37-49. Available from: https://bvsms.saude.gov.br/bvs/publicacoes/amamentacao_uso_medicamentos_outras_substancias_2ed icao.pdf

[68] Lexicomp. Amantadine: Drug information. Lexicomp 2020. Available from: https://www.uptodate.com/contents/amantadine-drug-information?search=amantadine&source =panel_search_result&selectedTitle=1~68&usage_type=panel&kp_tab=drug_general&display_rank= 1#F50642731

[69] Lexicomp. Rimantadine: Drug information. Lexicomp 2020. Available from: https://www.uptodate.com/contents/rimantadine-drug-information?search=rimantadina&source =panel_search_result&selectedTitle=1~16&usage_type=panel&kp_tab=drug_general&display_rank= 1

[70] Lexicomp. Olsetamivir: Drug information. Lexicomp 2020. Available from:

https://www.uptodate.com/contents/oseltamivir-drug-information?search=oseltamivir&source =search_result&selectedTitle=1~50&usage_type=panel&kp_tab=drug_general&display_rank=1#F204 099

[71] Lexicomp. Zanamivir: Drug information. Lexicomp 2020. Available from: https://www.uptodate.com/contents/zanamivir-drug-information?search=zanamivir&source =search_result&selectedTitle=1~26&usage_type=panel&kp_tab=drug_general&display_rank=1#F235 653

[72] Lexicomp. Quinine: Drug information. Lexicomp 2020. Available from: https://www.uptodate.com/contents/quinine-drug-information?search=quinina&source =panel_search_result&selectedTitle=1~95&usage_type=panel&kp_tab=drug_general&display_rank= 1#F3343867

[73] World Health Organization. Guidelines for the treatment of malaria 2015; (3): 285-99. Available from: https://apps.who.int/iris/bitstream/handle/10665/162441/ 9789241549127_eng.pdf;jsessionid=37BE3AA032C94476D 9E840753E2F25B0?sequence =1

[74] Daily J, Berghella V. Malaria in pregnancy: Prevention and treatment. Treatment: Antimalarial therapy 2020. Available from: https://www.uptodate.com/contents/malaria-in-pregnancy-prevent-on-and-treatment

[75] Hill J, Hoyt J, Eijk AM, *et al.* Factors Affecting the Delivery, Access, and Use of Interventions to Prevent Malaria in Pregnancy in Sub-Saharan Africa: A Systematic Review and Meta-Analysis. PLOS Medicine 2013; 10(7): 2-18. Available from: https://journals.plos.org/plosmedicine/article?id=10.1371/journal.pmed.1001488 [PMID: 1001488]

[76] Intermittent preventive treatment in pregnancy (IPTp). World Health Organization: World Health Organization WHO Recommendations 2019. Available from: https://www.who.int/malaria/areas/preventive_therapies/pregnancy/en/

[77] Carvalho FR, Dart JK, Ophthalmol AJ, *et al.* Drugs for Parasitic Infections. Drugs for Parasitic Infections. 2013; 11: 21-9. Available from: https://www.uab.edu/medicine/gorgas/images/docs/syllabus/2015/03_Parasites/RxParasitesMedicalLet ter2013.pdf

[78] Ryan ET. Mass drug administration for control of parasitic infections. Parasite targets for mass drug administration;[revised 16th Sep 2020; cited 22nd Jul 2020] 2020. Available from: https://www.uptodate.com/contents/mass-drug-administration-for-control-of-parasitic-infe ctions?search=ivermectina%20gravidez&source=search_result&selectedTitle=7~44&usage_type=defa ult&display_rank=6#H10826579

[79] Leder K. Anthelminthic therapies. Praziquantel 2020. Available from: https://www.uptodate.com/contents/mass-drug-administration-for-control-of- parasitic-infections?search=ivermectina%20gravidez&source=search_result&selectedTitle= 7~44&usage_type=default&display_rank=6#H10826579

[80] Drugs and Lactation Database (LactMed): Ivermectin. National Library of Medicine (USA): Bethesda. Drug Levels and Effects: Summary of Use during Lactation 2018. Available from: https://www.ncbi.nlm.nih.gov/books/NBK501375/

CHAPTER 4

Treatment of Urinary Tract Infections in Pregnancy

Ayane Cristine Alves Sarmento, Antônio Carlos Queiroz de Aquino, Michelly Nóbrega Monteiro and **Iaponira da Silva Figueiredo Vidal***

Federal University of Rio Grande do Norte, Nilo Peçanha Av., 259, Natal, Brazil

Abstract: Among the infections that can affect women during pregnancy, about 10% are represented by urinary tract infections (UTI), which are the most common type of infection during pregnancy. Depending on the part of the urinary tract they affect, they are known as Cystitis and Asymptomatic Bacteriuria, when they occur in the lower tract, or pyelonephritis when the infection in the lower tract ascends. All clinical types of UTI can lead to serious maternal and fetal complications. Thus, differently to the non-pregnant patient, all UTIs during pregnancy, including those with asymptomatic infection, need treatment. When we identify more than one episode in the same pregnancy, prophylactic treatment is recommended.

Keywords: Antibiotics, Bacteriuria, Pregnancy, Pyelonephritis, Urinary tract infections.

BACKGROUND

UTIs are the second most frequent disease in pregnancy after anemia, and the most common type of infection throughout pregnancy [1]. Approximately 5-10% of women present some type of UTI in pregnancy, representing around 5% of all hospital admissions for these women [2].

Adaptive alterations that occur in the urinary tract of pregnant women predisposed to the development of the UTIs can be classified as asymptomatic or symptomatic. Asymptomatic bacteriuria is characterized as the isolation of bacteria in at least 1x105 colony-forming units per mL of cultured urine, in which there is a lack of signs or symptoms. Symptomatic UTIs are classified into lower tract (acute cystitis) or upper tract (acute pyelonephritis) infections [3]. Asymptomatic bacteriuria develops in 2–15% of pregnant women and is an

* **Corresponding author Iaponira da Silva Figueiredo Vidal:** Federal University of Rio Grande do Norte, Nilo Peçanha Av., 259, Natal, Brazil; Tel: +558432155969; E-mail: iaponiravidal277@gmail.com

important risk factor for developing symptomatic UTIs [4].

Asymptomatic bacteriuria and acute cystitis contribute considerably to an increase in the risk of developing pyelonephritis, and also may cause severe maternal and fetal complications, such as preterm labor, low birth weight, or maternal systemic infection. For this reason, these infections represent major diagnostic and therapeutic challenges [1].

PATHOGENESIS

Changes resulting from the adaptive mechanisms of the urogenital tract in pregnancy, such as dilation of the ureters, occur at the beginning of the seventh week of gestation and are provoked by smooth muscle relaxation stimulated by progesterone, while mechanical compression of the enlarged pregnant uterus also contributes to the development of hydronephrosis [5]. This occurs especially in the right kidney, and an increase in plasma volume can decrease urine concentration and increase bladder volume. The factors mentioned previously cause urinary stasis and vesicoureteral reflux. As well as this, changes in pH and urine osmolality, such as glycosuria and aminoaciduria provoked in pregnancy, further promote bacterial growth and urgent treatment of the UTI [6].

RISK FACTORS

Low socioeconomic status and illiteracy are pointed out by several studies [7 - 9] as risk factors for asymptomatic bacteriuria, as these women tend to start prenatal follow-up late, due to less access to information regarding its importance. The shortage of urine tests and improper handling of UTI in these pregnant women end up adding to the predisposing factors that cause UTI in these patients who start prenatal care late. It should also be noted that ASB is the main predisposing factor that causes symptomatic bacteriuria. The most common anatomical conditions which predispose to pyelonephritis are hydroureter and hydronephrosis, and vesicoureteral reflux is the main functional alteration. In addition to these, we should also mention anemia, insulin resistance, diabetes, and the presence of infectious diseases that require metabolic adaptations. Countless researches have shown that UTI in pregnancy is related to an increased risk of premature birth, and therefore it is proposed that screening for UTI at the first prenatal consultation and during the second and third trimester of pregnancy may inhibit the manifestation of this pregnancy complication [7 - 9].

MICROBIOLOGY

The most frequent pathogenic in pregnancy is *Escherichia coli*, responsible for up to 86% of UTI cases, as well as other microorganisms such as *Streptococcus agalactiae* (26%), *Staphylococcus spp* (24%), *Klebsiella spp* (16%), *Proteus spp* (9%), *Pseudomonas spp* (6%), *Enterococcus spp* (4%), and *Enterobacter spp* (3%) are all frequently associated. Other pathogens are associated with a lower frequency and lower severity [10 - 13].

CLASSIFICATION OF UTIS

Urinary tract infections during pregnancy are classified as asymptomatic or symptomatic. They are asymptomatic bacteriuria, acute cystitis and acute pyelonephritis [14].

Asymptomatic Bacteriuria

It is said that the patient has Asymptomatic Bacteriuria when there is the presence or growth in the urine of 1 or more specified bacterial species ($\geq$105 CFU/mL or $\geq$108 CFU/L) [4]. If microorganisms, such as lactobacillus bacteria, which are not typical uropathogens, are isolated, treatment should be reserved for patients in whom the organism grows as a single isolate in consecutive cultures [15].

Prior evaluation methods such as rod, enzymatic screening, reagent strip or interleukin-8 in terms of sensitivity and specificity are not as accurate as urine culture and should not be used for the diagnosis of ASB in pregnant women [16]. The diagnosis of asymptomatic bacteriuria needs to be confirmed by certain methods; usually it is done using the culture of a carefully collected urine sample to minimize contamination by external agents. For this, it is recommended that the patient performs the collection after the local cleaning of the urethral meatus and the surrounding mucosa and the first stream of urine is discarded [17]. There is insufficient data to support a recommendation for or against repeated screening during pregnancy for a patient, even with a negative initial screening culture or after an initial episode of treated ASB [18].

The treatment of asymptomatic bacteriuria is performed with an antibiotic adapted to the susceptibility pattern of the isolated organism, which is usually available at the time of diagnosis. Beta-lactams, nitrofurantoin and phosphomycin are some of the potential options. The choice of antimicrobial agent should be made carefully, while also taking into account the safety and continuity of the pregnancy [17 - 22]. Currently, it is not known what is the ideal duration for the treatment of asymptomatic bacteriuria. The short-term evidence-based therapy is the most widely accepted approach, recommending a treatment regimen of three to seven days [23, 24]. The treatment scheme can be observed in Table **1**.

Table 1. Antibiotics indicated for the treatment of ASB and cystitis in pregnant women.

Antibiotic	Dose	Duration	Notes
Amoxicillin	500mg orally 8/8 hours or 875 orally every 12 hours	5 to 7 days	The resistance to gram-negative pathogens may be a limitation for its use
Amoxicillin -clavulonate	500mg orally 8/8 hours or 875 orally every 12 hours	5 to 7 days	
Cefpodoxime	100mg orally 12/ 12 hours	5 to 7 days	
Cephalexin	250 to 500mg orally 6/6 hours	5 to 7 days	
Fosfomycin	3g orally in a single dose		Due to its nephrotoxicity, do not use doses higher than the recommended therapies. Do not use if the patient is suspected of having pyelonephritis.
Nitrofurantoin	100mg orally 12/12 hours	5 to 7 days	Due to its nephrotoxicity, do not use doses higher than the recommended therapies. Do not use if the patient is suspected of having pyelonephritis. Avoid use during the first quarter and in the long term
Trimethoprim-sulfamethoxazole	800 / 160mg (loading dose) 12/12 hours	3 days	Avoid use during the first quarter and in the long term

Acute Cystitis

Dysuria is one of the main symptoms of acute cystitis in pregnant women. The doctor should evaluate these symptoms, as these findings are commonly found in pregnant women with a normal physiological profile, and who do not present with cystitis [25].

If pregnant women present new dysuria, urinalysis and urine culture should be done. It is prudent to use a quantitative count of ≥ 103 cfu/ml in a symptomatic pregnant woman as an indicator of symptomatic UI. If bacteria that are not typically uropathogenic are isolated, the diagnosis for cystitis is made if they are isolated at high bacterial counts (≥ 105 cfu/mL) [26].

Care for acute cystitis in pregnant women includes empirical antibiotic therapy, which should be adapted to the results of the urine culture, and then follow up cultures to confirm the absence of bacteria in the urine. There is no ideal duration of treatment for acute cystitis, and it is uncertain when it should end. Treatment should be completed when there is clinical improvement and no more bacteria in the urine. As in cases of asymptomatic bacteriuria, short courses of antibiotics are advisable to minimize possible antimicrobial exposure to the fetus [27 - 29]. The treatment scheme can be observed in Table **1**.

Acute Pyelonephritis

Acute pyelonephritis is a pathology that affects the superior urinary tract. Flank pain, fever (>38°C), nausea and/or costovertebral angle sensitivity are typical symptoms of acute pyelonephritis in pregnant women and can be observed in non-pregnant women. Pyuria is a typical finding, and there is not always the presence of dysuria. In addition to these symptoms, a potential manifestation includes hematological changes such as anemia and thrombocytopenia. Pyelonephritis can cause medical and obstetric complications in pregnant women. It is estimated that 20% of pregnant women with grave pyelonephritis may present complications that range from septic shock to Acute Respiratory Discomfort Syndrome (ARDS) [30, 31].

For pregnant women with fever and/or back pain, symptomatic for pyelonephritis, it is essential that this is considered as a differential diagnosis: intraamniotic infection, with or without premature labor. Some researchers have questioned the value of obtaining routine blood cultures in pregnant women with pyelonephritis, and although data on the impact of blood cultures on results are limited, obtaining blood cultures from those with signs of sepsis or serious underlying medical conditions, such as diabetes, is recommended [32, 33].

Serum lactate level is a test that can be used to investigate pregnant women with sepsis and is a good marker for the disease. Imaging tests are not routinely used for the diagnosis of pyelonephritis. However, in severe patients who also have symptoms of kidney colic or lithiasis, immunosuppression, a history of previous urological surgery, diabetes, repeated episodes of pyelonephritis, or urosepsis, kidney imaging tests might be useful in investigating complications due to pyelonephritis. In pregnant women, kidney ultrasonography is the most widely used imaging test because it prevents exposure to contrast and radiation [34].

Hospitalization for parenteral antibiotics is the most widely used treatment for acute pyelonephritis; however, antibiotic therapy can be converted to an oral regimen. For this, it is important to observe the susceptibility profile of the isolated organism after the clinical evolution of the patient. Broad spectrum parenteral beta-lactam drugs are preferred for the initial empiric treatment of pyelonephritis. It is up to the doctor or the infection control committee to select the most suitable beta-lactam for the treatment of pyelonephritis in pregnant women. Other classes of antimicrobials such as fluoroquinolones and aminoglycosides are also used for the treatment of pyelonephritis in non-pregnant patients and should be avoided in pregnant women, as there is higher toxicity compared to other classes of pyelonephritis [29, 30].

As with non-pregnant patients with pyelonephritis, normally, after 24 to 48 hours of antibiotic therapy, pyelonephritis is overcome. If the patient is afebrile for 48 hours, she can make use of oral therapy, always guided by the results of urine culture and be discharged from the hospital to complete home treatment with oral antibiotics for 10-14 days. Oral antibiotic therapy options are limited, including beta-lactams, and in the second trimester of pregnancy, the use of sulfamethoxazole+trimethoprim. The use of phosphomycin and nitrofurantoin is not indicated for the treatment of pyelonephritis due to low tissue concentration [30].

There is no recommendation for termination of pregnancy in patients with pyelonephritis. When birth is indicated, it is recommended to wait for the patient to reach an afebrile clinical state, as long as there is clinical safety for the pregnant woman and the fetus. If it is not possible and there is a possibility of preterm delivery, the use of tocolines and steroids is indicated to try to prolong the time of pregnancy [31]. The treatment scheme can be observed in Table **2**.

Table **2**. Antibiotics indicated for the treatment of pyelonephritis in pregnant women.

Antibiotic	Dose/Interval
Mild to moderate pyelonephritis	
Ampicillin + **Gentamicin** **Aztreonam** **Cefepime** **Ceftriaxone**	1-2g 6/6 hours 1.5mg/kg 8/8 hours 1g 8/8 hours 1g 12/12 hours 1g 24/24 hours
Severity pyelonephritis	
Ertapenem **Doripenem** **Meropenem** **Piperacilin-tazobactam**	1g 24/24 hours 500mg 8/8 hours 1g 8/8 hours 3.375g every 6 hours

ANTIBIOTIC SAFETY IN PREGNANCY

There are not many studies on the safety of new antibiotics in the treatment of pregnancy complications, as these drugs may cause damage to the fetus. Thus, there is little direct information about the safety of many newer antibiotics in pregnancy, and concern about the use of certain antibiotics generally derives from indirect evidence (*e.g.*, animal studies) or observational studies that may have numerous confounders [35].

Overall, the safest course is to use the antibiotics that have well- established safety profiles in pregnancy and limit the use of antibiotics of potential concern to cases in which no safer alternative exists. It is generally accepted that penicillins (with or without beta-lactamase inhibitors) and cephalosporins are safe in pregnancy. Some animal studies have shown that carbapenems lead to adverse fetal effects, this includes the use of imipenem-cylastatin, therefore the preferred carbapenems for use during pregnancy are meropenem, doripenem and ertapenem. Nitrofurantoin is frequently used during pregnancy, although some potential concerns exist [36, 37]. Studies suggest a risk of fetal or newborn hemolytic anemia induced by the use of nitrofurantoin, especially in neonates with G6PD enzyme deficiency [18].

The use of trimethoprim-sulfamethoxazole is typically limited to mid- pregnancy, avoiding the first trimester and near term. However, with this there is no proven teratogenic effect in humans. The use of sulfonamides in the last days of pregnancy should be avoided, as there is a possibility of displacement of indirect bilirubin from the plasma of the newborn to the nuclei of the base, which may have an increased risk of developing a brain injury known as kernicterus. Although kernicterus is related solely to sulfonamide exposure, this manifestation has never been reported *via* intrauterine. The use of aminoglycosides in pregnancy has been associated with a higher risk of ototoxicity after long periods of fetal exposure, therefore, the use of this class of antimicrobials should be avoided, unless there is intolerance or resistance of other antimicrobials that justifies its use. The use of tetracycline after the 16th week of pregnancy is not indicated, as it is associated with the depigmentation of the child's decidual dentition. Also, gentamycin can cause damage to the vestibulocochlear nerve in the fetus [18], and fluoroquinolones are generally not used during pregnancy [38, 39].

ANTIBIOTICS IN BREASTFEEDING

Breast milk is essential for the health of the child because it provides nutrients and immune active substances. As well as this, it favors the mother-child affective relationship and the child's development, from a cognitive and psychomotor point of view. Despite the advantages of breast milk, there are occasions when the health professional should consider the risk/benefit of drug therapy in the breastfeeding mother. However, it is important to remember that, the mammary alveolar epithelium functions as an almost impermeable barrier [41, 42].

Most drugs pass into breast milk in small quantities; and even when present in milk, these drugs may or may not be absorbed into the gastrointestinal tract of the infant. When maternal illness requires treatment with medications incompatible with breastfeeding, this method of feeding should be stopped. Antibiotics are often prescribed during breastfeeding, for short periods, thus reducing the risk for the infant. The main concern is the change in the intestinal flora of the child, leading to diarrhea and moniliasis and possible interference in the interpretation of the result from cultures of the infant [41, 42] (Table **3**).

Table 3. Guidance for the use of antibiotics in breastfeeding.

Antibiotics in Breastfeeding	
Penicillins (amoxicillin, ampicillin, cloxacillin, floxacillin, oxacillin, among others)	They reach low concentrations in breast milk. They are usually prescribed to treat infections in newborns and infants. Side effects are rarely observed, and can occasionally cause allergic reactions, such as rash. In this case, there must be replacement of the antimicrobial, guidance for the mother to maintain breastfeeding, and avoidance of the use of the drug in the child in the future.
Cephalosporins (cefaclor, cefadroxil, cefazolin, cefepime, cefazolin, among others)	It offers little risk to the infant due to the strong link to maternal plasma proteins, causing a small amount of the drug to pass into the milk. There could be the possibility of modification of the intestinal flora, direct effects on the child, and interference in the interpretation of the result of cultures. Moniliasis and diarrhea can be observed in the infant.
Aminoglycosides (amikacin, spectinomycin, streptomycin, kanamycin, netylmycin, tobramycin)	Can easily appear in the breast milk, however, absorption in the infant's gastrointestinal tract is negligible. Although safe breastfeeding can occur, there are changes in the infant's intestinal flora.
Sulphonamides (sulfacetamide, sulfadiazine, Silver sulfadiazine, sulfamethoxazole + trimetropin, among others)	The excretion of these drugs in the infant varies widely. It can interfere with the connection of bilirubin with albumin, increasing the risk of Kernicterus. The use must be judicious in the preterm newborn in the first month of life and children with hyperbilirubinemia and/or with Glucose-6-phosphate dehydrogenase (G-6-PD) defect. It should be noted that jaundice, rash, and diarrhea present in the infant. Preference should be given to short-acting and intermediate sulfonamides.
Quinolones (ofloxacin, ciprofloxacin, levofloxacin, moxifloxacin, norfloxacin, among others)	These are not usually recommended in pediatric patients due to the potential risk of affecting growth cartilage development. However, studies and recent reviews have highlighted the safety of quinolones in the pediatric age group. The dose excreted in breast milk is too low to cause arthropathy.

(Table 3) contd.....

Antibiotics in Breastfeeding	
Macrolides **(azithromycin, clarithomycin,** **erythromycin, among others)**	Most are compatible with breastfeeding. Caution is needed in the use of Telithromycin and Dirithromycin, as there are no safety data for use during the lactation period.
Beta-lactams **(aztreonam, ertapenem,** **imipenem, Meropenem)**	Most are compatible with breastfeeding, except Meropenem, as there are no safety data for use during the lactation period. It is observed that excretion into breast milk is likely due to low molecular weight.

NON ANTIBIOTIC MEASURES

The discovery of safe treatment alternatives to the use of antibiotics to prevent and treat UTIs in pregnancy is of paramount importance, since antimicrobial resistance currently represents a constant danger [43]. The guidelines for the European Association of Urology (EAU) responding to studied hygiene habits, pointed out that there is no known association of these habits with the incidence of UTIs, although, some studies provide evidence that this association exists. Increased sexual activity (3/4 times a week) was also indicated as a factor that increases the risk of UTIs. But, the habit of washing the genital area and voiding the bladder after intercourse was demonstrated to have a defensive action for UTIs [44, 45].

Clinical trials were performed [45, 46] to evaluate the positive effectiveness of cranberry juice to prevent the appearance of UTIs in pregnant women. These studies pointed out that cranberry juice has a possible effect for this purpose. However, the studies presented some limitations which brought uncertainty into the effectiveness of this treatment. One of these limitations was the high volume of juice that is necessary to be ingested (240 ml and 250 ml) [46]. The researches presented a high amount of abandonment, principally because of gastrointestinal disturbances, which ended up limiting its use for reasons of acceptability. For this reason, there is the necessity to explore a standardized formulation of cranberries, such as tablets and capsules, thus helping to improve adherence and tolerability of this treatment [47, 48].

Investigating the role of immunization to lower the recurrence of UTIs in pregnant women demonstrated positive outcomes. However, important limitations were observed, for example, not having a control group, lack of blinding and unclear risk of bias. Therefore, the use of immunization to prevent UTIs in pregnancy requires more analysis to determine its usefulness in practice [43].

The use of ascorbic acid once a day can be favorable, principally in regions with a large incidence of UTIs and antimicrobial resistance. Although the study results were promising, the realization of new research to intensify the previous data should be suggested. In general, it is necessary to perform new researches to intensify the evidences using upgraded study design and more efficient reporting of clinical trials to indicate what options can be recommended in practice [49].

RECURRENT UTIS

The definition of Recurrent UTIs (rUTIs) consists of the recurrence of simple and/or complicated UTIs, with a repetition of at least 3 UTIs in a year or 2 in the last 6 months. While, UTIs encompass both cystitis and pyelonephritis, recurrent pyelonephritis should be considered a more problematic etiology [50].

For diagnosis of UTI, routine exams, such as cystoscopy and imaging, are not recommended, because the diagnostic yield is low. The UTI must be verified by urine culture. However, in atypical cases (renal calculi or outflow obstruction), they should be performed quickly [51, 52].

According to systematic reviews realized by the Cochrane database, for the prophylaxis, antimicrobials may be indicated in extended low-dose for continued periods (3 to 6 months) or as post intercourse prophylaxis [54]. Regimens incorporate nitrofurantoin 50 mg or 100 mg once daily, fosfomycin trometamol at 3 g every ten days, and throughout the pregnancy cephalexin 125 mg or 250 mg or cefaclor 250 mg once daily [55]. When behavioral alteration and non-antimicrobial options have no affect, these regimes should be indicated. The prophylaxis postcoital can be indicated in women with a history of frequent UTIs before the start of pregnancy [56].

PREVENTION OF RECURRENT UTIS

A separate issue is the management of pregnant women with a past of rUTIs before pregnancy, which is generally associated with sexual intercourse. The preferred regimen of prophylaxis postcoital in pregnant women is a single post-coital dose of either cephalexin (250 mg) or nitrofurantoin (50 mg) [57, 58].

CONCLUSIONS

Diverse non-antimicrobial treatments suggested for rUTIs exist. Despite the existence of powerful screening methods, UTIs still continue to be one among the most frequent diseases present in pregnant women from many different countries. Difficulties in diagnosis can occur since the symptoms may be nonspecific, and are similar to healthy pregnant women. Unlike the general population, asymptomatic UTIs in pregnancy women necessitate valid treatment from reliable international organizations. Initial diagnosis and satisfactory treatment of asymptomatic UTIs enable a significant decrease in maternal and fetal aggravation. Many of the drugs can be safely used during pregnancy. The most frequent pathogens in UTIs present sensitivity, and can be treated during the first trimester. The urine culture test is the principal method of the diagnosis and should be realized as a routine maternal procedure starting from the first trimester and for all pregnant women.

CONSENT FOR PUBLICATION

Not applicable.

CONFLICT OF INTEREST

The authors declare no conflict of interest, financial or otherwise.

ACKNOWLEDGEMENTS

Declared none.

REFERENCES

[1]   Amiri M, Lavasani Z, Norouzirad R, *et al.* Prevalence of urinary tract infection among pregnant women and its complications in their newborns during the birth in the hospitals of Dezful City, Iran, 2012–2013. Iran Red Crescent Med J 2015; 17(8): e26946.
[http://dx.doi.org/10.5812/ircmj.26946] [PMID: 26430526]

[2]   Souza RB, Trevisol DJ, Schuelter-Trevisol F. Bacterial sensitivity to fosfomycin in pregnant women with urinary infection. Braz J Infect Dis 2015; 19(3): 319-23.
[http://dx.doi.org/10.1016/j.bjid.2014.12.009] [PMID: 25626961]

[3]   Bahadi A, El Kabbaj D, Elfazazi H, *et al.* Urinary tract infection in pregnancy. Saudi J Kidney Dis Transpl 2010; 21(2): 342-4.
[PMID: 20228527]

[4]   Nicolle LE, Gupta K, Bradley SF, *et al.* Clinical practice guideline for the management of asymptomatic bacteriuria: 2019 update by the infectious diseases society of America. Clin Infect Dis 2019; 68(10): e83-e110.
[http://dx.doi.org/10.1093/cid/ciz021]

[5]   Jeyabalan A, Lain KY. Anatomic and functional changes of the upper urinary tract during pregnancy. Urol Clin North Am 2007; 34(1): 1-6.
[http://dx.doi.org/10.1016/j.ucl.2006.10.008] [PMID: 17145354]

[6]   Ipe DS, Horton E, Ulett GC. The basics of bacteriuria: strategies of microbes for persistence in urine. Front Cell Infect Microbiol 2016; 6: 14.
[http://dx.doi.org/10.3389/fcimb.2016.00014] [PMID: 26904513]

[7]   Bahadi A, El Kabbaj D, Elfazazi H, *et al.* Urinary tract infection in pregnancy. Saudi J Kidney Dis Transpl 2010; 21(2): 342-4.
[PMID: 20228527]

[8]   Sheiner E, Mazor-Drey E, Levy AJ. Asymptomatic bacteriuria during pregnancy. Maternal-Fetal and Neonatal Medicine 2019; 22: 423-7.
[http://dx.doi.org/10.1080/14767050802360783]

[9]   Celen S, Oruç AS, Karayalçin R, *et al.* Asymptomatic bacteriuria and antibacterial susceptibility patterns in an obstetric population. ISRN Obstet Gynecol 2011; 2011: 721872.
[http://dx.doi.org/10.5402/2011/721872] [PMID: 21647231]

[10]   Ipe DS, Sundac L, Benjamin WH Jr, Moore KH, Ulett GC. Asymptomatic bacteriuria: prevalence rates of causal microorganisms, etiology of infection in different patient populations, and recent advances in molecular detection. FEMS Microbiol Lett 2013; 346(1): 1-10.
[http://dx.doi.org/10.1111/1574-6968.12204] [PMID: 23808987]

[11]   Izadi B, Rostami-Far Z, Jalilian N, *et al.* Urinary tract infection (UTI) as a risk factor of severe preeclampsia. Glob J Health Sci 2016; 8: 543-6.
[http://dx.doi.org/10.5539/gjhs.v8n11p77]

[12]   Rezavand N, Veisi F, Zangane M, Amini R, Almasi A. Association between asymptomatic bacteriuria and pre-eclampsia. Glob J Health Sci 2015; 8(7): 235-9.
[http://dx.doi.org/10.5539/gjhs.v8n7p235] [PMID: 26925912]

[13]   Easter SR, Cantonwine DE, Zera CA, Lim KH, Parry SI, McElrath TF. Urinary tract infection during pregnancy, angiogenic factor profiles, and risk of preeclampsia. Am J Obstet 2016; 214: 387. e1-e7.
[http://dx.doi.org/10.1016/j.ajog.2015.09.101]

[14]   Sobel JD, Kaye D. Urinary tract infections. In: Mandell GL, Bennett J, Dolin R, Eds. Mandell, Douglas, and Bennett's Principles and practice of infectious diseases, 7. Philadelphia: Elsevier 2010; 1: p. 957.
[http://dx.doi.org/10.1016/B978-0-443-06839-3.00069-2]

[15]   Schneeberger C, van den Heuvel ER, Erwich JJ, Stolk RP, Visser CE, Geerlings SE. Contamination rates of three urine-sampling methods to assess bacteriuria in pregnant women. Obstet Gynecol 2013; 121(2 Pt 1): 299-305.
[http://dx.doi.org/10.1097/AOG.0b013e31827e8cfe] [PMID: 23344279]

[16]   Baerheim A, Digranes A, Hunskaar S. Evaluation of urine sampling technique: bacterial contamination of samples from women students. Br J Gen Pract 1992; 42(359): 241-3.
[PMID: 1419246]

[17]   Lin K, Fajardo K. Screening for asymptomatic bacteriuria in adults: evidence for the U.S. Preventive Services Task Force reaffirmation recommendation statement. Ann Intern Med 2008; 149(1): W20-4.
[http://dx.doi.org/10.7326/0003-4819-149-1-200807010-00009-w1] [PMID: 18591632]

[18]   Smaill FM, Vazquez JC. Antibiotics for asymptomatic bacteriuria in pregnancy. Cochrane Database Syst Rev 2019; 2019(11): CD000490.
[http://dx.doi.org/10.1002/14651858.cd000490.pub4] [PMID: 31765489]

[19]   Gratacós E, Torres PJ, Vila J, Alonso PL, Cararach V. Screening and treatment of asymptomatic bacteriuria in pregnancy prevent pyelonephritis. J Infect Dis 1994; 169(6): 1390-2.
[http://dx.doi.org/10.1093/infdis/169.6.1390] [PMID: 8195624]

[20]   Zinner SH, Kass EH. Long-term (10 to 14 years) follow-up of bacteriuria of pregnancy. N Engl J Med 1971; 285(15): 820-4.
[http://dx.doi.org/10.1056/NEJM197110072851502] [PMID: 4936826]

[21]   Widmer M, Lopez I, Gülmezoglu AM, *et al.* Duration of treatment for asymptomatic bacteriuria during pregnancy. Cochrane Database Syst Ver 2015; CD000491..
[http://dx.doi.org/10.1002/14651858.CD000491.pub3]

[22]   Reeves DS. Treatment of bacteriuria in pregnancy with single dose fosfomycin trometamol: a review. Infection 1992; 20 (Suppl. 4): S313-6.
[http://dx.doi.org/10.1007/BF01710022] [PMID: 1294525]

[23]   Whalley PJ, Cunningham FG. Short-term *versus* continuous antimicrobial therapy for asymptomatic bacteriuria in pregnancy. Obstet Gynecol 1977; 49(3): 262-5.
[PMID: 320525]

[24]   Widmer M, Gülmezoglu AM, Mignini L, Roganti A. Duration of treatment for asymptomatic bacteriuria during pregnancy. Cochrane Database Syst Rev 2011; (12): CD000491.
[http://dx.doi.org/10.1002/14651858.CD000491.pub2] [PMID: 22161364]

[25]   Stamm WE, Counts GW, Running KR, Fihn S, Turck M, Holmes KK. Diagnosis of coliform infection in acutely dysuric women. N Engl J Med 1982; 307(8): 463-8.
[http://dx.doi.org/10.1056/NEJM198208193070802] [PMID: 7099208]

[26]   Hooton TM, Roberts PL, Cox ME, Stapleton AE. Voided midstream urine culture and acute cystitis in premenopausal women. N Engl J Med 2013; 369(20): 1883-91.
[http://dx.doi.org/10.1056/NEJMoa1302186] [PMID: 24224622]

[27]   Gupta K, Hooton TM, Naber KG, *et al.* International clinical practice guidelines for the treatment of acute uncomplicated cystitis and pyelonephritis in women: A 2010 update by the Infectious Diseases Society of America and the European Society for Microbiology and Infectious Diseases. Clin Infect Dis 2011; 52(5): e103-20.
[http://dx.doi.org/10.1093/cid/ciq257] [PMID: 21292654]

[28]   Vazquez JC, Abalos E. Treatments for symptomatic urinary tract infections during pregnancy. Cochrane Database Syst Ver 2011; CD002256.
[http://dx.doi.org/10.1002/14651858.CD002256.pub2]

[29]   Lutters M, Vogt-Ferrier NB. Antibiotic duration for treating uncomplicated, symptomatic lower urinary tract infections in elderly women. Cochrane Database Syst Ver 2008; CD001535.
[http://dx.doi.org/10.1002/14651858.CD001535.pub2]

[30]   Hill JB, Sheffield JS, McIntire DD, Wendel GD Jr. Acute pyelonephritis in pregnancy. Obstet Gynecol 2005; 105(1): 18-23.
[http://dx.doi.org/10.1097/01.AOG.0000149154.96285.a0] [PMID: 15625136]

[31]   Wing DA, Fassett MJ, Getahun D. Acute pyelonephritis in pregnancy: an 18-year retrospective analysis. Am J Obstet Gynecol 2014; 210(3): 219.e1-6.
[http://dx.doi.org/10.1016/j.ajog.2013.10.006] [PMID: 24100227]

[32]   Cunningham FG, Lucas MJ. Urinary tract infections complicating pregnancy. Baillieres Clin Obstet Gynaecol 1994; 8(2): 353-73.
[http://dx.doi.org/10.1016/S0950-3552(05)80325-6] [PMID: 7924012]

[33]   Gomi H, Goto Y, Laopaiboon M, *et al.* Routine blood cultures in the management of pyelonephritis in pregnancy for improving outcomes. Cochrane Database Syst Ver 2015; CD009216.
[http://dx.doi.org/10.1002/14651858.CD009216.pub2]

[34]   Albright CM, Ali TN, Lopes V, Rouse DJ, Anderson BL. Lactic acid measurement to identify risk of morbidity from sepsis in pregnancy. Am J Perinatol 2015; 32(5): 481-6.
[PMID: 25486284]

[35]   American College of Obstetricians and Gynecologists. Antimicrobial therapy for obstetric patients. ACOG Educ Bull 1998; 245. Washington, DC.

[36]   Kahlmeter G. Prevalence and antimicrobial susceptibility of pathogens in uncomplicated cystitis in Europe. The ECO.SENS study. Int J Antimicrob Agents 2003; 22 (Suppl. 2): 49-52.
[http://dx.doi.org/10.1016/S0924-8579(03)00229-2] [PMID: 14527771]

[37]   Naber KG, Schito G, Botto H, Palou J, Mazzei T. Surveillance study in Europe and Brazil on clinical aspects and Antimicrobial Resistance Epidemiology in Females with Cystitis (ARESC): implications for empiric therapy. Eur Urol 2008; 54(5): 1164-75.
[http://dx.doi.org/10.1016/j.eururo.2008.05.010] [PMID: 18511178]

[38]   Zhanel GG, Hisanaga TL, Laing NM, *et al.* Antibiotic resistance in *Escherichia coli* outpatient urinary isolates: final results from the North American Urinary Tract Infection Collaborative Alliance (NAUTICA). Int J Antimicrob Agents 2006; 27(6): 468-75.
[http://dx.doi.org/10.1016/j.ijantimicag.2006.02.009] [PMID: 16713191]

[39]   Harris RE, Gilstrap LC III. Prevention of recurrent pyelonephritis during pregnancy. Obstet Gynecol 1974; 44(5): 637-41.
        [PMID: 4419749]

[40]   Berlin C, Briggs G. Drugs and chemicals in human milk. Seminars in fetal and neonatal medicine 2005; 10: 149-59.

[41]   Anderson P, Pochop C, Manoguerra A. Adverse drug reactions in breastfed infants: Less than imagined. Clin Pediatr 2003; 42: 325-40.

[42]   DRUGSAFETY. Drug safety during pregnancy and breastfeeding 2020. Disponível em: https://www.perinatology.com/exposures/druglist.htm

[43]   Ghouri F, Hollywood A, Ryan K. A systematic review of non-antibiotic measures for the prevention of urinary tract infections in pregnancy. BMC Pregnancy Childbirth 2018; 18(1): 99.
        [http://dx.doi.org/10.1186/s12884-018-1732-2] [PMID: 29653573]

[44]   Bonkat G, Pickard R, Bartoletti R, *et al.* Guideline: urological infections. Eur Assoc Urol 2017.

[45]   Wing DA, Rumney PJ, Preslicka CW, Chung JH. Daily cranberry juice for the prevention of asymptomatic bacteriuria in pregnancy: a randomized, controlled pilot study. J Urol 2008; 180(4): 1367-72.
        [http://dx.doi.org/10.1016/j.juro.2008.06.016] [PMID: 18707726]

[46]   Essadi F, Elmehashi MO. Efficacy of cranberry juice for the prevention of urinary tract infections in pregnancy [abstract]. Poster Session J Matern Fetal Neonatal Med 2010; 23(1): 378.
        [http://dx.doi.org/10.3109/ 14767051003802503]

[47]   Dugoua J-J, Seely D, Perri D, Mills E, Koren G. Safety and efficacy of cranberry (vaccinium macrocarpon) during pregnancy and lactation. Can J Clin Pharmacol 2008; 15(1): e80-6.
        [PMID: 18204103]

[48]   Heitmann K, Nordeng H, Holst L. Pregnancy outcome after use of cranberry in pregnancy--the Norwegian Mother and Child Cohort Study. BMC Complement Altern Med 2013; 13: 345.
        [http://dx.doi.org/10.1186/1472-6882-13-345] [PMID: 24314317]

[49]   Ochoa-Brust GJ, Fernández AR, Villanueva-Ruiz GJ, Velasco R, Trujillo-Hernández B, Vásquez C. Daily intake of 100 mg ascorbic acid as urinary tract infection prophylactic agent during pregnancy. Acta Obstet Gynecol Scand 2007; 86(7): 783-7.
        [http://dx.doi.org/10.1080/00016340701273189] [PMID: 17611821]

[50]   Bonkat G, Pickard R, Bartoletti R, *et al.* EUA guideline on urological infections. European Association of Urology 2017.

[51]   Hooton TM. Prevention of recurrent urogenital tract infections in adult women.EAU/International Consultation on Urological Infections. The Netherlands: European Association of Urology 2010.

[52]   Beerepoot MA, Geerlings SE, van Haarst EP, van Charante NM, ter Riet G. Nonantibiotic prophylaxis for recurrent urinary tract infections: a systematic review and meta-analysis of randomized controlled trials. J Urol 2013; 190(6): 1981-9.
        [http://dx.doi.org/10.1016/j.juro.2013.04.142] [PMID: 23867306]

[53]   Wagenlehner FM, Vahlensieck W, Bauer HW, Weidner W, Piechota HJ, Naber KG. Prevention of recurrent urinary tract infections. Minerva Urol Nefrol 2013; 65(1): 9-20.
        [PMID: 23538307]

[54]   Albert X, Huertas I, Pereiró II, Sanfélix J, Gosalbes V, Perrota C. Antibiotics for preventing recurrent urinary tract infection in non-pregnant women. Cochrane Database Syst Rev 2004; (3): : CD001209.
        [http://dx.doi.org/10.1002/14651858.CD001209.pub2] [PMID: 15266443]

[55]   Hooton TM. Recurrent urinary tract infection in women. Int J Antimicrob Agents 2001; 17(4): 259-68.
        [http://dx.doi.org/10.1016/S0924-8579(00)00350-2] [PMID: 11295405]

[56] Pfau A, Sacks TG. Effective prophylaxis for recurrent urinary tract infections during pregnancy. Clin Infect Dis 1992; 14(4): 810-4.
[http://dx.doi.org/10.1093/clinids/14.4.810] [PMID: 1576275]

[57] Keating GM. Fosfomycin trometamol: a review of its use as a single-dose oral treatment for patients with acute lower urinary tract infections and pregnant women with asymptomatic bacteriuria. Drugs 2013; 73(17): 1951-66.
[http://dx.doi.org/10.1007/s40265-013-0143-y] [PMID: 24202878]

[58] Crider KS, Cleves MA, Reefhuis J, Berry RJ, Hobbs CA, Hu DJ. Antibacterial medication use during pregnancy and risk of birth defects: National Birth Defects Prevention Study. Arch Pediatr Adolesc Med 2009; 163(11): 978-85.
[http://dx.doi.org/10.1001/archpediatrics.2009.188] [PMID: 19884587]

Anti-infective Agents for Sexually Transmitted Infections in Pregnancy

Ana Paula Costa[*], **Ayane Cristina Sarmento**, **Maria da Conceição Cornetta** and **Ana Katherine Gonçalves**

Department of Postgraduate Program in Health Sciences, Federal University of Rio Grande do Norte, Natal, Brazil

Abstract: During pregnancy, the occurrence of Sexually Transmitted Infections (STI) is a problem aggravated by the presence of the fetus, which presents difficulties in the use of certain drugs and the physiological adaptations of this phase in the pregnancy-puerperal cycle. The World Health Organization (WHO) estimates that 448 million new STIs worldwide occur each year, of which the most frequent are associated with human papillomavirus (HPV), *Chlamydia trachomatis*, *Neisseria gonorrhoeae*.

Keywords: *Chlamydia trachomatis*, HSV, HTLV, HPV, *Neisseria gonorrhoeae*, Pregnant Woman, Sexually Transmitted Infections, Syphilis, ZIKV.

BACKGROUND

The STIs have been found responsible for a high number of pathologies associated with the pregnancy-puerperal cycle [1]. Laboratory studies suggest that pregnancy interferes with the maternal defense mechanism by immunosuppression [2]. The Center for Disease Control and Prevention (CDC), pointed out, wich STIs during pregnancy, like chlamydia, gonorrhea, syphilis, HIV and hepatitis B were reported on women ages 15 to 24 years and the presence was verified in the first prenatal visit [3, 4].

The increase in certain STIs could in some cases be justified by local anatomical and functional changes that occur in pregnant women. The hyperproliferation and engorgement (edema and increased blood flow) of the vaginal wall, the increase in glycogen of the epithelium and the significant decrease in vaginal pH are some of the factors that could facilitate the onset and spread of infections [5].

[*] **Corresponding author Ana Paula Ferreira Costa:** Department of Postgraduate Program in Health Sciences, Federal University of Rio Grande do Norte, Natal, Brazil; Tel: +5584996391560; E-mail: ana-paula-rf@hotmail.com

During pregnancy, sexually transmitted infections can worsen the health of women and babies. Despite this, women remain underscreened for STIs during pregnancy [4]. This lack of oversight is detrimental to womens' and infants' health, and there is the risk to suffer more significant damage, that include premature birth, miscarriage, preterm labor and premature rupture of membranes [6].

VIRAL GENITAL INFECTIONS

Human Papillomavirus (HPV)

The HPV is the most common viral infection, especially, in young women of reproductive age. HPV is a DNA virus that infects basal epithelial cells. HPV type 16 and 18 are reported as the main risk factors of invasive cervical cancers [7], while others, like 6 and 11 have been associated with warts [8].

HPV detection increases with disease severity, with the percentage of positivity in cervical intraepithelial neoplasia 1 (CIN1) being at 50 –70%, CIN2 has (85%) positivity for HPV, and in CIN3 and invasive cervical cancer the positivity rises to between (90% - 100%) [9].

Physiological changes during pregnancy modulate the functions of the immune system, and usually, this changes the HPV behavior [10], which is also acting on the persistence of the virus in the cervical epithelial cells, stimulating the infection. In pregnancy, the increased mucus in the cervical glands and the proliferation of basal and parabasal layers of stratified squamous epithelium among others changes, become the pregnancy more susceptible to the impact of the infection [11].

The prevalence of HPV in pregnant women is controversial. Some studies have not shown statistical significance in pregnant and not-pregnant women. However, data in the literature, state that the prevalence of HPV ranges from 5.5 to 65% [12]. The different types of HPV are responsible for different pathologies of the cervix, so genotyping is important during pregnancy. The literature points out that high concentrations of estrogen and progesterone in the blood of pregnant women and in the cervical epithelial cells activate the expression of the initial HPV genes [13].

Most HPV infections are resolved spontaneously [14]. However, during pregnancy, HPV infection may persist and regress after delivery [15]. HPV has uniqueness in relation to long-term latency, episodic detectability and genital and intrauterine localization. *In vitro* studies and animal models have shown that HPV can replicate in trophoblasts, leading to (1) inhibition of blastocyst formation; (2) endometrial implantation; and (3) embryonic cell apoptosis. In addition, the HPV-trophoblast interaction could trigger hypersensitivity to bacterial infections, leading to complications in pregnancy, such as pre-eclampsia or premature labor [16].

The methods to diagnose HPV infection are a Pap smear, which is a screening test. A positive test requires further confirmatory tests like colposcopy, cervical biopsy, and DNA tests like polymerase chain reaction (PCR). The colposcopy allows for the examination of the cervix and vagina; the cervical biopsy is a critical part with results that can show pre-cancer (dysplasia) or cancer; and the DNA test (PCR, Southern Blot Hybridization, In Situ Hybridization) for molecular detection of HPV.

Condyloma and injuries caused by HPV can be treated during pregnancy. The choice of the best treatment method depends on several factors, such as the number and extent of the lesions and the location affected. In the case of warts, for example, the laser is one of the best options, or if it is on the outside of the genital region, an acid can be applied, whereas for extensive lesions surgical ablation is more effective. These procedures are released at any stage of pregnancy. But, the ideal is that they are carried out until the 34th week, to guarantee a good healing before childbirth. Techniques contraindicated in pregnancy are electrocauterization, which stimulates uterine contraction; immunomodulators, which do not have studies that prove their effectiveness during pregnancy; and podophyllin, which can be toxic [17, 18].

Among the chemical agents, podophyllin and 5-fluorouracil, although commonly used in the treatment of condyloma, should not be administered to pregnant women due to the teratogenic effect. Trichloroacetic acid (80% to 90%), due to its good cure rates (50% -81%) and not being absorbed systemically, constitutes first-line therapy in pregnant women with small or few lesions. Imiquimod for the treatment of injuries in pregnant women is restricted to case reports and, therefore, its use is not allowed in these patients. The interferon has not been proven effective for this population with regard to the treatment of genital warts [17].

Herpes Simplex Vírus (HSV)

Herpes simplex virus (HSV) is a double-stranded DNA virus belonging to the Herpesviridae family. HSV exists as a subtype, HSV-1 and HSV-2, both of which cause infections [19]. Genital herpes is the predominant STI, which has assumed massive proportions, being the most common in developed and high-frequency countries in young women [20]. Highly prevalent in the population of pregnant women, the HSV, during pregnancy, has been associated with miscarriages, intrauterine growth retardation, preterm labor, and neonatal infections ranging from 30% to 50% for infections which occur late in pregnancy due to insufficient antibody development to suppress viral replication before delivery [21].

HSV genital infections are often subclinical and, even if asymptomatic, their signs and symptoms may be non-specific. Clinical symptoms in the external genitalia and cervix such as blisters and ulceration, vulvar pain, dysuria, vaginal discharge, local lymphadenopathy, vesicular and ulcerative lesions in the inner thigh, buttocks and perineum can be observed [22]. Disseminated HSV infection can be severe and life-threatening, involving the central nervous system (CNS) and visceral involvement. In pregnancy, it is rare to spread from the primary infection, but if it occurs during the second or third trimester, there is a higher risk of transmitting the virus to the baby. The decrease of innate and adaptive immunity in the mother can be associated with the HSV infection on pregnancy [23].

All suspected HSV infections should be confirmed by viral or serological tests. Viral detection techniques are by viral culture and the detection of HSV antigen by the polymerase chain reaction (PCR) enables the differentiation between HSV-1 and HSV-2 by providing higher sensitivity. Antibody detection techniques include the use of laboratory-based serological tests to detect the presence of antibodies to HSV-1 or HSV-2. The HSV infection should be confirmed serologically or with viral culture, being, the latter, the preferred diagnostic test for patients seeking medical treatment for genital ulcers or other mucocutaneous lesions, besides it allows for the differentiation of virus type [21, 24].

Acyclovir treatment can be used in certain situations: the oral and intravenous forms reduce injury time, although it is not approved for current use in pregnancy, it has been used to treat severe HSV infections in the gestational period without observed fetal impairment. Given the severe complications of the first HSV infection in the third trimester of pregnancy, intravenous acyclovir therapy may be indicated [21]

Human Immunodeficiency Virus (HIV)

The human immunodeficiency virus (HIV) causes Acquired Immunodeficiency Syndrome (AIDS), which appeared in the United States in 1981, causing damage to the immune system of infected individuals. The virus destroys CD4 + T cells, making the individual immunodeficient [25]. In pregnancy, unlike other viral infections, maternal HIV infection is not associated with congenital anomalies and/or adverse effects on the miscarriage rate [26]. Vertical transmission that can occur in the uterus, during delivery, or in the postpartum period through breastfeeding is the primary concern. Postpartum risk is directly linked to the HIV viral load in maternal plasma, the higher the burden, the greater the risks [27]. However, vertical transmission can be avoided, using strategies such as antiretroviral therapy (ART), cesarean section and access to milk powder, and transmission varies from less than 2% in the developed world to more than 30% in the developing world [28].

Observational studies have shown that HIV infection is associated with increased miscarriages, stillbirths, perinatal and infant mortality, and intrauterine growth retardation, among others. Infection can reduce fertility, causing HIV-infected women to have lower pregnancy rates than uninfected women [29]. Access to prenatal care promotes the survival of both the woman and the fetus. From the available resources and the individual needs of women, a multidisciplinary team can improve care. In HIV-positive women pre-gestational counseling can optimize medical care and minimize adverse outcomes [30].

Most postpartum complications include postpartum sepsis, infected episiotomies, condylomata acuminata en masse, urinary tract infections, pneumonia, fever, tuberculosis and unusual infections [31]. So, the laboratory investigations, in addition to routine pregnancy tests, should include liver function tests, complete blood count, plasma RNA viral load, and infection screening for sexually transmitted diseases [32].

The diagnosis of HIV infection is made from blood collection or oral fluid. Laboratory tests and rapid tests detect antibodies to HIV in about 30 minutes. Tests for HIV infection can be divided into four groups:

✓ Detection of antibodies;

✓ Detection of antigens;

✓ Viral culture;

✓ Amplification of the virus genome.

The techniques routinely used for the diagnosis of HIV infection are based on the detection of antibodies against the virus. These techniques present excellent results and are less expensive, and are considered the best choice for an initial screening. However, they detect the host's response to the virus, not the virus itself. The other three techniques directly detect the virus or its particles. They are less frequently used routinely, being applied in specific situations, such as uncertain or doubtful serological tests, laboratory follow-up of patients and the measurement of viral load for treatment control. Each technique will now be explained separately [33].

ART can reduce vertical transmission from viral load reduction in prepartum, pre-exposure and post-exposure prophylaxis of the child [34]. Therefore, for the prevention of perinatal transmission of HIV, intrapartum and infantile, antiretroviral prophylaxis is recommended. Combined therapeutic regimens are considered the standard for the treatment of HIV infection and the prevention of perinatal transmission. Clinical Trials show that the administration of zidovudine (AZT, ZDV) during pregnancy and the child could reduce the risk of perinatal transmission by almost 70% [35].

Preferred regimens have demonstrated efficacy, safety, and ease of use. The schemes include the following:

• Tenofovir disoproxil fumarate with emtricitabine (TDF/FTC co-formulated) or tenofovir disoproxil fumarate with lamivudine (3TC) taken once daily;

• Abacavir with lamivudine (ABC/3TC) taken once daily; avoid combination with ritonavir-boosted atazanavir if the pretreatment HIV viral load exceeds 100,000 copies/mL [36].

Protease Inhibitor

• Atazanavir (ATV) plus ritonavir(RTV): ATV 300 mg plus RTV 100 mg PO as a single daily dose; some experts increase ATV/RTV dose to 400/100 mg daily during second and third trimester; manufacturer recommends dose increase in pregnancy if combined with tenofovir or H2 blocker in treatment-experienced patients and with efavirenz in treatment-naive patients [37];

• Darunavir (DRV) 600 mg plus 100 mg RTV taken twice daily: Once-daily dosing achieves low darunavir trough in pregnancy and should not be used, especially in treatment-experienced patients [38].

Integrase Inhibitor Regimen

• Raltegravir (RAL) 400 mg taken twice daily: No data on the use of once-daily raltegravir 600-mg HD formulation in pregnancy; a rapid reduction in viral load potentially useful if presented late in pregnancy; hepatic enzyme elevation has occurred when used in late pregnancy [39].

Human T-Lymphotropic Virus (HTLV)

Human T-lymphotropic virus (HTLV) was the first human retrovirus to be studied and classified into two groups: HTLV-1 and HTLV-2. Two new viruses, HTLV-3 and HTLV-4, but, these viruses were not associated with human disease and transmission between humans has not been demonstrated [40].

The majority of those infected with HTLV are asymptomatic, with only 10% presenting characteristic symptoms. HTLV-1 is highly pathogenic, carriers develop serious clinical manifestations such as adult T-cell leukemia/lymphoma (HTLV), HTLV-associated myelopathy/tropical spastic paraparesis (HAM/TSP) and infectious dermatitis [41]. HTLV-2 is less pathogenic than HTLV-1, although there are reports of possible association with neurological diseases, such as HAM/TSP [3]. There is no effective antiviral treatment for HTLV-1/2 and the drugs currently available have not shown satisfactory results [42].

HTLV-1/2 infection, as well as other sexually transmitted diseases, occurs through unprotected sex, there is also the occurrence of vertical transmission, mainly through breastfeeding, parenteral transmission, blood transfusion and sharing of needles and syringes by users of intravenous drugs [43]. The efficient transmission of HTLV, occurs through a mechanism known as a virological synapse, where the virus passes from an infected cell to a new host cell, in which the virus subverts the normal T-cell physiology. Whereas HTLV- 1 infects mobile cells (lymphocytes), the virological synapse maximizes transmission efficiency and limits virus exposure to host defense mechanisms [44].

Vertical transmission of HTLV-1/2 could occur during the intrauterine period or during delivery, but it is through breastfeeding that most of its transmission occurs, with HTLV-infected cells entering the baby's body orally. Prenatal screening for HTLV should be implemented and combined with advice for HIV-positive mothers regarding transmission through breastfeeding. Non-breastfeeding as well as the use of pasteurized milk has been successfully applied to prevent HTLV infection [43].

The diagnosis of HTLV infection is based on the serological detection of antibodies specific to antigenic components of the different portions of the virus (core and envelope). Immunoenzymatic tests, with duplicate serum samples, have the advantage of being simple and of high sensitivity. Samples that present reagent results are submitted to confirmatory tests, such as Western blot and/or PCR [45]. Western blotting assays used the total viral lysate plus recombinant immunodominant epitopes corresponding to the N-terminal portion of the HTLV-I/II transmembrane (gp21) protein (r21-e and GD21-I peptides) as the antigen. These tests have high sensitivity to detect antibodies against the recombinant epitope. In PCR, consensual primers can be used, which aim at the differential diagnosis of the infection caused by HTLV-1/2, or to use specific, unique primers of HTLV-1 or HTLV-2 [46].

There is no specific intervention for acute or chronic (HTLV) infection. The treatment is directed according to the disease related to the virus. Mogamulizumab, a humanized anti-CCR4 monoclonal antibody defucosylated CCR4 is used in patients diagnosed with aggressive types of ACL (acute or lymphoma). Other regimens include interferon alpha, topoisomerase inhibitors, zidovudine plus interferon alpha and monoclonal antibodies against IL-2R and other receptors on ATL cells [47].

Hepatitis B Virus (HBV)

The hepatitis B virus (HBV) Infection is a serious public health problem worldwide and a significant cause of chronic hepatitis, cirrhosis, and hepatocellular carcinoma (HCC). In the past, it was believed that the infection was transmitted only by blood or contaminated instruments such as syringes and needles. Today, it is known that heterosexual transmission accounts for 25% of HBV cases, being numerically more relevant than homosexual relationships [48, 49].

Viral hepatitis during pregnancy is associated with a high risk of maternal complications, causing fetal and neonatal hepatitis and has been reported as a leading cause of maternal mortality [50]. Vertical transmission can occur from the transplacental transmission of HBV in utero, natal transmission during delivery or postnatal transmission during care of the infant or through breast milk [51].

In prenatal care, all efforts should be directed to the serological identification of the pregnant woman with HBV. Since prenatal screening is not possible, it is advisable to perform it in all pregnant women at the time of delivery [52].

It has not been proven that the cesarean section reduces HBV vertical transmission, so the delivery route, in these cases, is the one that obstetric evolution determines. The usual procedures for a vaginal delivery are the same, except for the episiotomy, which should be performed only in cases where the indication is indisputable. As a rule, clamping of the umbilical cord, and aspiration of the upper airways, oropharynx and the infant's stomach in a gentle and atraumatic manner are essential [53].

Clinically, acute B-hepatitis is characterized by increased hepatic enzymes (transaminases, alkaline phosphatase, gamma-glutamyltransferase) and the appearance of some specific markers of infection. During the clinical expression phase of HBV, laboratory tests are expected to confirm the following biological markers: virus surface antigen (HBsAg), antigen "e" (HBeAg), and anti-HBcAg and anti-HBeAg antibodies. Anti-HBsAg is expressed late, usually six months after the phase of clinical manifestations in patients with a favorable prognosis, representing the natural history of the disease [54].

If the non-HBV pregnant woman is exposed to a sufficient risk of contamination, passive immunotherapy with specific human gammaglobulin at a dose of 0.06 ml/kg body weight is indicated, and the treatment is repeated four weeks later. Both passive and active immunotherapy (a vaccine made with recombinant DNA techniques) can be used safely during pregnancy, but this period should not be confused with the choice to start a vaccine program, however safe it may be [55].

Considering the prevention of HBV, the newborn should receive active immunotherapy (vaccine) and passive (specific immunoglobulin against HBV), preferably in the first 12 hours of life. These applications are administered in the form of intramuscular injections. The vaccination schedule should continue to be programmed for the second dose in the first month of life, and the third dose in the sixth month. The effectiveness of the vaccine can reach 85%, whereas the combination with the immunoglobulin has a greater efficacy which reaches 95% [56].

Hepatitis C Virus (HCV)

HCV causes hepatitis of type acute and chronic. Acute HCV refers to the premier six months of infection later in contact with the virus, and has no symptoms in 75% of patients. If the symptoms manifest, it can be observed abdominal discomfort, vomiting, anorexia, jaundice, or pain [57]. The other 55% to 85% of patients with acute HCV continue to harbor the virus after 6 months of exposure, constituting a diagnosis of chronicity of the disease, that despite is frequently asymptomatic; can originate gradual liver harm, causing grave consequences to the patient [58].

The transmission of HCV occurs principally over contact percutaneous with blood infected. The main reason the occurs contamination of HCV in children is the vertical transmission [59]. One-third to one-half of vertical transmission can become in utero previous to the last month of gestation, whereas the is believed the other cases occur in the last month of gestation or delivery [60].

Studies suggest that HCV is related to results negative in gestation. Newborns to HCV-infected women have a more significant likelihood to presented low weight, be small for gestational age, need the support of ventilation, and be admitted to the neonatal intensive care unit [61]. Newborns have a greater predisposition to present alimentation difficulty or some type of adverse neurological outcome (brachial plexus damage, cephalohematoma, fetal suffering, feeding difficulty, intraventricular bleeding, and neonatal seizures). Another antepartum complication associated with HCV infection is intrahepatic cholestasis of pregnancy (ICP); the frequency of this illness is considerably bigger among pregnant women with HCV [62].

HCV infection is diagnosed is based on the detection of anti-HCV antibodies and HCV RNA. Anti-HCV antibodies expand during an acute infection-usually between 2 and 6 months contact previous -and continue throughout life. Accompaniment for HCV consists of tests for anti-HCV antibody. A positive result demonstrates actual infection (acute or chronic), the previous infection remedied, or a false-positive and will be accompanied by a nucleic acid test for HCV RNA [58, 63].

The existence of HCV RNA in the blood, express active infection; and can be identified from one to three weeks after contact. If HCV viremia is detected in patients with results negative for HCV RNA in the last six months, acute HCV condition is determined [64]. In cases with no preceding diagnostics that confirm infection by hepatitis C, for both anti-HCV antibodies and HCV RNA, it becomes impractical to differentiate acute from chronic HCV. Whether antibody testing returns negative in a patient that may have do exposed to HCV in the last six months, the HCV RNA test should be realized, as the seroconversion cannot have happened yet [65]. All pregnant women diagnosed with HCV infection should be forwarded to a hepatologist or infectologist qualified in the treatment of hepatitis to were observed long-term [66].

The treatment initially standardized for chronic HCV included interferon (PegIFN)-a and ribavirin, however, (PegIFN-a/ribavirin) these drugs presented important side effects, as well the risk of grave infection, hemolytic anemia, depression, and an influenza syndrome [67]. After that, direct-acting antiviral (DAA) pharmacies were liberated, remodel the treatment of HCV. These medications presented minor side effects than interferon-based regimens and obtain led to a bigger standard variable rate [68].

At present, the antiviral therapies indicate for the treatment of HCV are not approved for use in pregnancy. Ribavirin is contraindicated as of its association with embryocidal and/or teratogenic effects in all animal species studied. Malformations of the gastrointestinal tract, skull, palate, jaw, limbs, skeleton, and eye have been observed in animal models. Also, due the ribavirin persists in non-plasma compartments for up to six months, the US Food and Drug Administration (FDA) attention that pregnancy should be avoided in women, too as in female partners of male patients taking ribavirin until six months after concluding the treatment [65, 69].

Studies of second-generation DAAs in pregnant women are limited: the information in human are unsatisfactory; thus, security information comes only from animal research. For this reason, no DAA has been authorized for the treatment of HCV infection in pregnancy [70].

ZIKA VIRUS (ZIKV)

Belonging to the *Flaviviridae* family, the ZIKA is constituted a single-stranded RNA [71]. It was discovered in 1947 in samples of rhesus febris monkey and Aedes africanus mosquitoes in Uganda's Zika Forest. ZIKV is widespread throughout Africa, Asia, and Oceania, being first discovered in humans outside Africa and Asia in the year 2007. In Brazil, the first case of local transmission of the virus was in May 2015 [72].

Similar to other infections, caused by viruses belonging to the Flaviviridae family, ZIKV infection in humans occurs from the entry of the virus into the skin cells through cellular receptors, allowing the virus to migrate to the lymph nodes and bloodstream [73]. Transmission occurs from the mosquito bite, mainly of the genus Aedes, including Ae. aegypti, Ae. africanus, and Ae. albopictus. Ae. aegypti is the main vector in Asia and was the primary suspect vector in outbreaks in South America. Aedes mosquitoes are distributed globally with native habits of warm tropical and subtropical regions [74]. Other non-vectors of Zika virus transmission include congenital [75], perinatal [76] and sexual transmission [77].

In humans, this disease is often asymptomatic in 80% of cases [73]. When symptoms manifest, they are typically mild and nonspecific, and similarities to other arbovirus infections (*e.g.*, dengue and chikungunya viruses) may confound the diagnosis. Symptoms commonly reported include pruritic (with spontaneous resolution) rash, fever (37.4 ° C - 38.0 ° C), arthralgia, myalgia, fatigue, headache, and conjunctivitis. Symptoms disappear within 2 weeks; reports of greater persistence are rare [78].

Sexual transmission is possible from genital, oral, and anal intercourse through the semen and/or infected female genital tract, occurring until 44 days after the outset of symptoms. Intrauterine transmission was discovered from the zika virus RNA by reverse transcription (RT -PCR) in the amniotic fluid of pregnant women with manifestations of ZIKV all along pregnancy where they gave birth to infants with microcephaly [79]. Was described presence the ZIKV RNA in tissues of stillborn fetuses, women affected in pregnancy, and in brains of babies born alive with microcephaly. It was also well-defined the possible intrapartum transmission: Viral RNA was identified in breast milk, although neonatal transmission over breastfeeding has not yet been reported. The care of maternal-fetal transmission of the virus depends on the prevention of mosquito bites and the practice of safe sex [80].

The diagnosis of ZIKV consists of the molecular (RT-PCR) detection of RNA from the zika virus in the acute phase of the disease. Blood and urine are the samples of choice, and plasma or serum samples may also be used [81]. Total blood tests that detect the RNA of the ZIKV for a long time are considered the test of choice. Serology consists of the identification of precise IgM by ELISA, which detects IgM antibodies from 4 to 5 days and until 12 weeks or more after the onset of symptoms. As it does not yet exist specialized antiviral treatment available for pregnant women, for now, symptom relief is the standard treatment. If the symptoms are uncomfortable, the use of antipyretics in pain control and fever, are indicated [82].

BACTERIAL GENITAL INFECTIONS

Neisseria Gonorrhoeae

Gonorrhea is a second sexually transmitted infection most commonly reported in all the world, caused by etiological agent *Neisseria gonorrhoeae* [83].

The infection may involve several mucous membranes in the female genital tract, including the urethra, cervix, uterine tubes, Bartholin and Skene glands, the anorectal canal, as well as extragenital sites, such as the abdominal cavity, pharynx, and conjunctiva [5].

The prevalence of the disease in pregnancy varies according to the population studied, with rates ranging from 0.5 to 7%, which may cause complications for both mother and fetus [84]. Pregnancy can significantly alter the evolution of gonococcal infection, which can entirely be asymptomatic, as in the vast majority of cases, causing only vaginal discharge and dysuria, and in some more severe cases, the onset of disseminated gonococcal disease occurring in the second or third arthritis, with mono- or polyarticular arthritis being the most frequent manifestation. Generally, the infection is accompanied by malaise, fever, and rash [85].

The occurrence of ascending uterine infection is rare, although it may occur in the first trimester, causing septic spontaneous abortion. Not only this, but if this increase comes later, it may cause chorioamnionitis, premature breaking of the membranes and preterm birth, or neonatal infection [86].

Molecular biology methods (PCR and hybrid capture) are the most suitable. These can be performed both on endocervical material and on urine samples. The diagnosis of gonococcus can also be achieved by gonococcal culture in a selective medium (Thayer-Martin), from endocervical specimens or by staining of these samples by Gram, although the sensitivity of the latter technique in women is only around 50% [56].

The treatment of the pregnant woman should be:

1 – Erythromycin - 500 mg orally 6/6 hs for 10 days

2 – Ampicillin PLUS (3.5g orally a single dose) + Probenecid (1g orally a single dose)

Chlamydia Trachomatis (CT)

The CT is an obligate intracellular bacterium that has various serotypes, among them that provoke lymphogranuloma venereum. *C. trachomatis* is the genital infection most common infectious disease reported to state health departments, principally among sexually active adolescents and young adults [87].

Although transmission to newborns over vaginal birth can cause conjunctivitis and pneumonitis, exist uncertainty about other adverse effects of CT infection all along the pregnancy. Some evidence showed that this infection may give negative complications, such as premature breaking of membranes, preterm birth, and low birth weight. The CT infection is also involved in postabortal, post-cesarean section, and postpartum maternal infections [88, 89]. The Centers for Disease Control and Prevention recommend monitoring on the first prenatal consultation and over in the third trimester for pregnant than 25 years old or those who have new or various sex partners. Due to the high risk of repetition, in women who have initial positive cultures or for those at high risk, screening must be repeated in the third trimester [90 - 93].

The diagnosis of chlamydial infection is usually made using serological methods, like ELISA. These methods are less sensitive than culture-based methods but have a rapid turnaround time and present lower requirements, making them more attractive as a point-of-care assay. Nucleic acid amplification tests (NAATs), inclusive PCR, are highly precise compared with culture and maintain high specificity [56].

Treatment of pregnant women diagnosed with CT is mandatory and significantly reduces the risk of obstetric complications without apparent harm.

Chlamydia trachomatis: Recommended Regimen treatment

1 – Azithromycin - 1g orally in a single dose

2 – Erytromicyn 500 mg - orally 6/6 hs for 7 days

3 – Amoxicillin 500 mg - orally 8/8 hs for 7 days

Syphilis

Caused by the spirochete *Treponema pallidum* (TP), syphilis is a sexually transmitted disease, and is a systemic infectious disease which provides a considerable demand to public health services all the world. The WHO estimates indicate that the worldwide occurrence of this disease reaches 12 million new cases annually, more frequently in developing countries [94].

Three stages of the disease are described: primary, secondary and tertiary syphilis (Table **1**). Immunomodulation verified during pregnancy undoubtedly also contributes to the polymorphism of syphilitic lesions in this period. Other factors such as the virulence of the infecting strain, the form of contamination, or if it is a reinfection, also influence the innumerable ways in which the disease manifests itself [95, 96] (Table **1**).

Table 1. Clinical Stage of Syphilis.

Stage	Period	Symptoms
Primary	21 days after infection	Painless ulcer in genitals, skin and mouth
Secondary	4 - 8 weeks after first infection	Body rash, headache, fever and lymphadenopathy
Tertiary	1 - 10 years after initial infection	Aortic insufficiency, aortic aneurysm, tabes dorsalis, loss of cortical function and altered mental state
Latent		
Early	One year after cure of the primary or secondary injuries	Signs and symptoms commonly disappear
Late	Indefinite period	Cardiovascular syphilis, neurosyphilis and syphilitic meningitis

It is supposed that syphilis obtained in pregnancy pursue the sequential stages of the primary, secondary, and latent syphilis see in untreated, non-pregnant adult patients. When maternal infection is not treated, it can occur stillbirth, preterm birth and congenital infection in a portion of surviving newborns. Admitted that one-third of pregnancies are to result in second-trimester spontaneous abortion or perinatal death, one third in a congenitally infected infant, and one third in an uninfected infant [96 - 98].

The non-treponemal screening tests include the VDRL (Venereal Disease Research Laboratory), RPR (rapid plasma reagin), or ART (automated reagin test). Nontreponemal test antibody titers normally are associated with disease activity and will be reported with a quantitative titer. Treponemal-specific tests include fluorescent treponemal antibody absorption test (FTA-ABS) or Treponema pallidum particle agglutination (TP-PA), and are fundamental to certify the diagnosis of syphilis after a positive nontreponemal test. Nontreponemal screening during pregnancy is recommended in the first prenatal visit, and again in the third trimester, principally in high-risk populations [99].

The drug of preferred for the treatment of all stages of syphilis is the Penicillin G, in benzathine, aqueous procaine, or aqueous crystalline form, and is the only adequate treatment for the prevention of congenital syphilis in pregnant women. Erythromycin can be effective in the mother, but may not prevent congenital syphilis because of the variability of the transplacental passage of the antibiotic. For patients who have a penicillin allergy, Ceftriaxone may prove useful in adults as an alternative treatment; but it is important to highlight that there is insufficient information on its use in pregnant women [100]. The use of azithromycin in pregnant women allergic to penicillin still has not been satisfactorily evaluated [101]. Tetracyclines, inclusive doxycycline, commonly are not recommended during pregnancy, although, can be used for the treatment of syphilis in the non-pregnant woman, the use of this antibiotic can increase the risk of yellow-brown discoloration of the fetal deciduous teeth [102].

CONCLUSION

The STIs still represent an important public health concern, once these infections are considerably frequent during pregnancy, and many are correlate in adverse results among infected women and they are newborn [1 - 3].

In pregnancy, the physiological modifications that occur, provoke changes in the course of STDs leading to obstetrical and neonatal complications. The treatment must conserve the physical integrity of the mother and baby, excluded possible risks and complications, once these drugs presented inherent toxicity.

Education, information, screening, treatment, and prevention are considered essential factors of prenatal care for women at risk the contamination. All health professionals must know the guidelines for pregnant patients since the administration of STIs are frequently altered in pregnancy. Prevention and treatment of sexual partners also contribute considerably to the efficacy of these actions. Thus, the triage of STIs during prenatal care is essential for early diagnosis and improved therapy management.

CONSENT FOR PUBLICATION

Not applicable.

CONFLICT OF INTEREST

The authors declare no conflict of interest, financial or otherwise.

ACKNOWLEDGEMENTS

Declared none.

REFERENCES

[1]   Costa MC, Bornhausen Demarch E, Azulay DR, Périssé ARS, Dias MFRG, Nery JAC. Sexually transmitted diseases during pregnancy: a synthesis of particularities. An Bras Dermatol 2010; 85(6): 767-82.
        [http://dx.doi.org/10.1590/S0365-05962010000600002] [PMID: 21308300]

[2]   Suzuki K, Tomasi TB Jr. Immune responses during pregnancy. Evidence of suppressor cells for splenic antibody response. J Exp Med 1979; 150(4): 898-908.
        [http://dx.doi.org/10.1084/jem.150.4.898] [PMID: 159935]

[3]   Sexually transmitted disease surveillance 2011. Atlanta, GA: Author 2012.

[4]   Fontenot HB, George ER. Sexually transmitted infections in pregnancy. Nurs Womens Health 2014; 18(1): 67-72.
        [http://dx.doi.org/10.1111/1751-486X.12095] [PMID: 24548498]

[5]   Walker CK, Sweet RL. Gonorrhea infection in women: prevalence, effects, screening, and management. Int J Womens Health 2011; 3: 197-206.
        [PMID: 21845064]

[6]   STDs & pregnancy-CDC fact sheet. Atlanta, GA: Author 2013.

[7]   Doorbar J. The papillomavirus life cycle. J Clin Virol 2005; 32 (Suppl. 1): S7-S15.
        [http://dx.doi.org/10.1016/j.jcv.2004.12.006] [PMID: 15753007]

[8]   Hsueh P-R. Human papillomavirus, genital warts, and vaccines. J Microbiol Immunol Infect 2009; 42(2): 101-6.
        [PMID: 19597640]

[9]   Burd EM. Human papillomavirus and cervical cancer. Clin Microbiol Rev 2003; 16(1): 1-17.
        [http://dx.doi.org/10.1128/CMR.16.1.1-17.2003] [PMID: 12525422]

[10]   Domža G, Gudlevičienė Z, Didžiapetrienė J, *et al.* Human papillomavirus infection in pregnant women. Arch Gynecol Obstet 2011; 284(5): 1105-12.
        [http://dx.doi.org/10.1007/s00404-010-1787-4] [PMID: 21170544]

[11]   Stanley MA. Epithelial cell responses to infection with human papillomavirus. Clin Microbiol Rev 2012; 25(2): 215-22.
[http://dx.doi.org/10.1128/CMR.05028-11] [PMID: 22491770]

[12]   Medeiros LR, Ethur AB, Hilgert JB, *et al.* Vertical transmission of the human papillomavirus: a systematic quantitative review. Cad Saude Publica 2005; 21(4): 1006-15.
[http://dx.doi.org/10.1590/S0102-311X2005000400003] [PMID: 16021238]

[13]   Morales-Peza N, Auewarakul P, Juárez V, García-Carrancá A, Cid-Arregui A. *In vivo* tissue-specific regulation of the human papillomavirus type 18 early promoter by estrogen, progesterone, and their antagonists. Virology 2002; 294(1): 135-40.
[http://dx.doi.org/10.1006/viro.2001.1287] [PMID: 11886272]

[14]   Jalil EM, Bastos FI, Melli PP, *et al.* HPV clearance in postpartum period of HIV-positive and negative women: a prospective follow-up study. BMC Infect Dis 2013; 13: 564.
[http://dx.doi.org/10.1186/1471-2334-13-564] [PMID: 24289532]

[15]   García-Carrancá X, Drudis T, Cañadas MP, *et al.* Human Papillomavirus (HPV) infection in pregnant women and mother-to-child transmission of genital HPV genotypes: a prospective study in Spain. BMC Infect Dis 2009; 9: 74.
[http://dx.doi.org/10.1186/1471-2334-9-74] [PMID: 19473489]

[16]   Niyibizi J, Zanré N, Mayrand M-H, Trottier H. The association between adverse pregnancy outcomes and maternal human papillomavirus infection: a systematic review protocol. Syst Rev 2017; 6(1): 53.
[http://dx.doi.org/10.1186/s13643-017-0443-5] [PMID: 28284227]

[17]   Lacey CJ. Therapy for genital human papillomavirus-related disease. J Clin Virol 2005; 32 (Suppl. 1): S82-90.
[http://dx.doi.org/10.1016/j.jcv.2004.10.020] [PMID: 15753016]

[18]   Chuang LT, Temin S, Camacho R, *et al.* Management and Care of Women With Invasive Cervical Cancer: American Society of Clinical Oncology Resource-Stratified Clinical Practice Guideline. J Glob Oncol 2016; 2(5): 311-40.
[http://dx.doi.org/10.1200/JGO.2016.003954] [PMID: 28717717]

[19]   Kolokotronis A, Doumas S. Herpes simplex virus infection, with particular reference to the progression and complications of primary herpetic gingivostomatitis. Clin Microbiol Infect 2006; 12(3): 202-11.
[http://dx.doi.org/10.1111/j.1469-0691.2005.01336.x] [PMID: 16451405]

[20]   Jaishankar D, Shukla D. Genital Herpes: Insights into Sexually Transmitted Infectious Disease. Microb Cell 2016; 3(9): 438-50.
[http://dx.doi.org/10.15698/mic2016.09.528] [PMID: 28357380]

[21]   Straface G, Selmin A, Zanardo V, De Santis M, Ercoli A, Scambia G. Herpes simplex virus infection in pregnancy. Infect Dis Obstet Gynecol 2012; 2012: 385697.
[http://dx.doi.org/10.1155/2012/385697] [PMID: 22566740]

[22]   LeGoff J, Zanré H, Bélec L. Diagnosis of genital herpes simplex virus infection in the clinical laboratory. Virol J 2014; 11: 83.
[http://dx.doi.org/10.1186/1743-422X-11-83] [PMID: 24885431]

[23]   Hussain NY, Uriel A, Mammen C, Bonington A. Disseminated herpes simplex infection during pregnancy, rare but important to recognise. Qatar Med J 2014; 2014(1): 61-4.
[http://dx.doi.org/10.5339/qmj.2014.11] [PMID: 25320695]

[24]   Money D, Steben M. SOGC clinical practice guidelines: Guidelines for the management of herpes simplex virus in pregnancy. Number 208, June 2008. Int J Gynaecol Obstet 2009; 104(2): 167-71.
[http://dx.doi.org/10.1016/j.ijgo.2008.10.028] [PMID: 19241496]

[25]   Kumar P. Sexually transmitted disease: Acquired immune deficiency syndrome: A Review. J Appl Pharm Sci 2011; 01: 35-43.

[26]   Bucceri AM, Somigliana E, Matrone R, *et al.* Combination antiretroviral therapy in 100 HIV--infected pregnant women. Hum Reprod 2002; 17(2): 436-41.
        [http://dx.doi.org/10.1093/humrep/17.2.436] [PMID: 11821291]

[27]   John-Stewart G, Mbori-Ngacha D, Ekpini R, *et al.* Breast-feeding and Transmission of HIV-1. J Acquir Immune Defic Syndr 2004; 35(2): 196-202.
        [http://dx.doi.org/10.1097/00126334-200402010-00015] [PMID: 14722454]

[28]   Teasdale CA, Marais BJ, Abrams EJ. HIV: prevention of mother-to-child transmission. BMJ Clin Evid 2011; p. 0909.

[29]   Alemu FM, Yalew AW, Fantahun M, Ashu EE. Antiretroviral Therapy and Pregnancy Outcomes in Developing Countries: A Systematic Review. Int J MCH AIDS 2015; 3(1): 31-43.
        [PMID: 27621984]

[30]   Momplaisir FM, Brady KA, Fekete T, Thompson DR, Diez Roux A, Yehia BR. Time of HIV Diagnosis and Engagement in Prenatal Care Impact Virologic Outcomes of Pregnant Women with HIV. PLoS One 2015; 10(7): e0132262.
        [http://dx.doi.org/10.1371/journal.pone.0132262] [PMID: 26132142]

[31]   Ngonzi J, Bebell LM, Fajardo Y, *et al.* Incidence of postpartum infection, outcomes and associated risk factors at Mbarara regional referral hospital in Uganda. BMC Pregnancy Childbirth 2018; 18(1): 270.
        [http://dx.doi.org/10.1186/s12884-018-1891-1] [PMID: 29954356]

[32]   Gray GE, McIntyre JA. HIV and pregnancy. BMJ 2007; 334(7600): 950-3.
        [http://dx.doi.org/10.1136/bmj.39176.674977.AD] [PMID: 17478849]

[33]   Fearon M. The laboratory diagnosis of HIV infections. Can J Infect Dis Med Microbiol 2005; 16(1): 26-30.
        [http://dx.doi.org/10.1155/2005/515063] [PMID: 18159524]

[34]   Neubert J, Pfeffer M, Borkhardt A, *et al.* Risk adapted transmission prophylaxis to prevent vertical HIV-1 transmission: effectiveness and safety of an abbreviated regimen of postnatal oral zidovudine. BMC Pregnancy Childbirth 2013; 13: 22.
        [http://dx.doi.org/10.1186/1471-2393-13-22] [PMID: 23347580]

[35]   Hurst SA, Appelgren KE, Kourtis AP. Prevention of mother-to-child transmission of Human Immunodeficiency Virus Type 1 (HIV): the role of neonatal and infant prophylaxis. Expert Rev Anti Infect Ther 2015; 13(2): 169-81.
        [http://dx.doi.org/10.1586/14787210.2015.999667] [PMID: 25578882]

[36]   Guidelines for the Use of Antiretroviral Agents in HIV-1-Infected Adults and Adolescents. Department of Health and Human Services 2016.

[37]   Kreitchmann R, Best BM, Wang J, *et al.* Pharmacokinetics of an increased atazanavir dose with and without tenofovir during the third trimester of pregnancy. J Acquir Immune Defic Syndr 2013; 63(1): 59-66.
        [http://dx.doi.org/10.1097/QAI.0b013e318289b4d2] [PMID: 23392467]

[38]   Zorrilla CD, Wright R, Osiyemi OO, *et al.* Total and unbound darunavir pharmacokinetics in pregnant women infected with HIV-1: results of a study of darunavir/ritonavir 600/100 mg administered twice daily. HIV Med 2014; 15(1): 50-6.
        [http://dx.doi.org/10.1111/hiv.12047] [PMID: 23731450]

[39]   Watts DH, Stek A, Best BM, *et al.* Raltegravir pharmacokinetics during pregnancy. J Acquir Immune Defic Syndr 2014; 67(4): 375-81.
        [http://dx.doi.org/10.1097/QAI.0000000000000318] [PMID: 25162818]

[40]   Paiva A, Casseb J. Origin and prevalence of human T-lymphotropic virus type 1 (HTLV-1) and type 2 (HTLV-2) among indigenous populations in the Americas. Rev Inst Med Trop 2015; 57(1): 1-13.
        [http://dx.doi.org/10.1590/S0036-46652015000100001] [PMID: 25651320]

[41]   Caskey MF, Morgan DJ, Porto AF, *et al.* Clinical manifestations associated with HTLV type I infection: a cross-sectional study. AIDS Res Hum Retroviruses 2007; 23(3): 365-71.
        [http://dx.doi.org/10.1089/aid.2006.0140] [PMID: 17411369]

[42]   Nicolás D, Ambrosioni J, Paredes R, *et al.* Infection with human retroviruses other than HIV-1: HIV-2, HTLV-1, HTLV-2, HTLV-3 and HTLV-4. Expert Rev Anti Infect Ther 2015; 13(8): 947-63.
        [http://dx.doi.org/10.1586/14787210.2015.1056157] [PMID: 26112187]

[43]   Carneiro-Proietti AB, Amaranto-Damasio MS, Leal-Horiguchi CF, *et al.* Mother-to-child transmission of human T-cell lymphotropic viruses-1/2: What we know, and what are the gaps in understanding and preventing this route of infection. J Pediatric Infect Dis Soc 2014; 3 (Suppl. 1): S24-9.
        [http://dx.doi.org/10.1093/jpids/piu070] [PMID: 25232474]

[44]   Paiva A, Casseb J. Sexual transmission of human T-cell lymphotropic virus type 1. Rev Soc Bras Med Trop 2014; 47(3) Uberaba.

[45]   Olaleye OD, Ogunniyi A, Sheng ZJ, Li Z, Rasheed S. Detection of HTLV-I antibodies and DNA in blood sample of a patient with myelopathy in Nigeria. Rev Inst Med Trop 1998; 40(1): 55-7.
        [http://dx.doi.org/10.1590/S0036-46651998000100011] [PMID: 9713139]

[46]   Komurian-Pradel F, Pelloquin F, Sonoda S, Osame M, de The G. Geographical subtypes demonstrated by RFLP following PCR in the LTR region of HTLV-I. AIDS Res Hum Retroviruses 1992; 8(4): 429-34.
        [http://dx.doi.org/10.1089/aid.1992.8.429] [PMID: 1350915]

[47]   Sato T, Coler-Reilly ALG, Yagishita N, *et al.* Mogamulizumab (Anti-CCR4) in HTLV-1-Associated Myelopathy. N Engl J Med 2018; 378(6): 529-38.
        [http://dx.doi.org/10.1056/NEJMoa1704827] [PMID: 29414279]

[48]   Zhang SL, Yue YF, Bai GQ, Shi L, Jiang H. Mechanism of intrauterine infection of hepatitis B virus. World J Gastroenterol 2004; 10(3): 437-8.
        [http://dx.doi.org/10.3748/wjg.v10.i3.437] [PMID: 14760774]

[49]   Wright TL. Introduction to chronic hepatitis B infection. Am J Gastroenterol 2006; 101 (Suppl. 1): S1-6.
        [PMID: 16448446]

[50]   Elinav E, Ben-Dov IZ, Shapira Y, *et al.* Acute hepatitis A infection in pregnancy is associated with high rates of gestational complications and preterm labor. Gastroenterology 2006; 130(4): 1129-34.
        [http://dx.doi.org/10.1053/j.gastro.2006.01.007] [PMID: 16618407]

[51]   Tse KY, Ho LF, Lao T. The impact of maternal HBsAg carrier status on pregnancy outcomes: a case-control study. J Hepatol 2005; 43(5): 771-5.
        [http://dx.doi.org/10.1016/j.jhep.2005.05.023] [PMID: 16139923]

[52]   Mullick S, Watson-Jones D, Beksinska M, Mabey D. Sexually transmitted infections in pregnancy: prevalence, impact on pregnancy outcomes, and approach to treatment in developing countries. Sex Transm Infect 2005; 81(4): 294-302.
        [http://dx.doi.org/10.1136/sti.2002.004077] [PMID: 16061534]

[53]   Dafallah SE, El-Agib FH, Bushra GO. Maternal mortality in a teaching hospital in Sudan. Saudi Med J 2003; 24(4): 369-72.
        [PMID: 12754536]

[54]   Okoth F, Mbuthia J, Gatheru Z, *et al.* Seroprevalence of hepatitis B markers in pregnant women in Kenya. East Afr Med J 2006; 83(9): 485-93.
        [PMID: 17447350]

[55]   Bertolini DA, Pinho JRR, Saraceni CP, Moreira RC, Granato CFH, Carrilho FJ. Prevalence of serological markers of hepatitis B virus in pregnant women from Paraná State, Brazil. Braz J Med Biol Res 2006; 39(8): 1083-90.
        [http://dx.doi.org/10.1590/S0100-879X2006000800011] [PMID: 16906283]

[56]   Workowski KA, Berman S. Sexually transmitted diseases treatment guidelines, 2010. MMWR Recomm Rep 2010; 59(RR-12): 1-110.
[PMID: 21160459]

[57]   World Health Organization. Guidelines for the screening, care and treatment of persons with chronic hepatitis C infection. 2016.

[58]   Sangiovanni A, Prati GM, Fasani P, *et al.* The natural history of compensated cirrhosis due to hepatitis C virus: A 17-year cohort study of 214 patients. Hepatology 2006; 43(6): 1303-10.
[http://dx.doi.org/10.1002/hep.21176] [PMID: 16729298]

[59]   Gower E, Estes C, Blach S, Razavi-Shearer K, Razavi H. Global epidemiology and genotype distribution of the hepatitis C virus infection. J Hepatol 2014; 61(1) (Suppl.): S45-57.
[http://dx.doi.org/10.1016/j.jhep.2014.07.027] [PMID: 25086286]

[60]   Jhaveri R, Swamy GK. Hepatitis C virus in pregnancy and early childhood: current understanding and knowledge deficits. J Pediatric Infect Dis Soc 2014; 3 (Suppl. 1): S13-8.
[http://dx.doi.org/10.1093/jpids/piu045] [PMID: 25232471]

[61]   Pergam SA, Wang CC, Gardella CM, Sandison TG, Phipps WT, Hawes SE. Pregnancy complications associated with hepatitis C: data from a 2003-2005 Washington state birth cohort. Am J Obstet Gynecol 2008; 199(1): 38.e1-9.
[http://dx.doi.org/10.1016/j.ajog.2008.03.052] [PMID: 18486089]

[62]   Wijarnpreecha K, Thongprayoon C, Sanguankeo A, Upala S, Ungprasert P, Cheungpasitporn W. Hepatitis C infection and intrahepatic cholestasis of pregnancy: A systematic review and meta-analysis. Clin Res Hepatol Gastroenterol 2017; 41(1): 39-45.
[http://dx.doi.org/10.1016/j.clinre.2016.07.004] [PMID: 27542514]

[63]   Maheshwari A, Thuluvath PJ. Management of acute hepatitis C. Clin Liver Dis 2010; 14(1): 169-176, x.
[http://dx.doi.org/10.1016/j.cld.2009.11.007] [PMID: 20123448]

[64]   Workowski KA, Bolan GA. Sexually transmitted diseases treatment guidelines, 2015. MMWR Recomm Rep 2015; 64(RR-03): 1-137.
[PMID: 26042815]

[65]   Joint Panel From the American Association for the Study of Liver Diseases and the Infectious Diseases Society of America. Recommendations for testing, managing, and treating hepatitis C 2016.
http://www.hcvguidelines.org/

[66]   McIntyre PG, Tosh K, McGuire W. Caesarean section *versus* vaginal delivery for preventing mother to infant hepatitis C virus transmission. Cochrane Database Syst Rev 2006; 4(4): CD005546.
[http://dx.doi.org/10.1002/14651858.CD005546.pub2] [PMID: 17054264]

[67]   American College of Obstetricians and Gynecologists. ACOG Practice Bulletin No. 86: Viral hepatitis in pregnancy. Obstet Gynecol 2007; 110(4): 941-56.
[http://dx.doi.org/10.1097/01.AOG.0000263930.28382.2a] [PMID: 17906043]

[68]   US National Library of Medicine. Drug label information: Ribasphere-ribavirin tablet. DailyMed 2011.

[69]   US Food and Drug Administration. Pregnancy and lactation labeling (Drugs). Final Rule 2016.

[70]   Martinez Viedma MDP, Pickett BE. Characterizing the Different Effects of Zika Virus Infection in Placenta and Microglia Cells. Viruses 2018; 10(11): E649.
[http://dx.doi.org/10.3390/v10110649] [PMID: 30453684]

[71]   Mishra B, Behera B. The mysterious Zika virus: Adding to the tropical flavivirus mayhem. J Postgrad Med 2016; 62(4): 249-54.
[http://dx.doi.org/10.4103/0022-3859.191006] [PMID: 27763483]

[72]   Plourde AR, Bloch EM. A Literature Review of Zika Virus. Emerg Infect Dis 2016; 22(7): 1185-92.

[http://dx.doi.org/10.3201/eid2207.151990] [PMID: 27070380]

[73]   Boyer S, Calvez E, Chouin-Carneiro T, Diallo D, Failloux AB. An overview of mosquito vectors of Zika virus. Microbes Infect 2018; 20(11-12): 646-60.
       [http://dx.doi.org/10.1016/j.micinf.2018.01.006] [PMID: 29481868]

[74]   Oliveira Melo AS, Malinger G, Ximenes R, Szejnfeld PO, Alves Sampaio S, Bispo de Filippis AM. Zika virus intrauterine infection causes fetal brain abnormality and microcephaly: tip of the iceberg? Ultrasound Obstet Gynecol 2016; 47(1): 6-7.
       [http://dx.doi.org/10.1002/uog.15831] [PMID: 26731034]

[75]   Besnard M, Lastere S, Teissier A, Cao-Lormeau V, Musso D. Evidence of perinatal transmission of Zika virus, French Polynesia, December 2013 and February 2014. Euro Surveill 2014; 19(13): 20751.
       [http://dx.doi.org/10.2807/1560-7917.ES2014.19.13.20751] [PMID: 24721538]

[76]   Musso D, Roche C, Robin E, Nhan T, Teissier A, Cao-Lormeau VM. Potential sexual transmission of Zika virus. Emerg Infect Dis 2015; 21(2): 359-61.
       [http://dx.doi.org/10.3201/eid2102.141363] [PMID: 25625872]

[77]   Patterson J, Sammon M, Garg M. Dengue, Zika and Chikungunya: Emerging Arboviruses in the New World. West J Emerg Med 2016; 17(6): 671-9.
       [http://dx.doi.org/10.5811/westjem.2016.9.30904] [PMID: 27833670]

[78]   Counotte MJ, Kim CR, Wang J, *et al.* Sexual transmission of Zika virus and other flaviviruses: A living systematic review. PLoS Med 2018; 15(7): e1002611.
       [http://dx.doi.org/10.1371/journal.pmed.1002611] [PMID: 30040845]

[79]   Citil Dogan A, Wayne S, Bauer S, *et al.* The Zika virus and pregnancy: evidence, management, and prevention. J Matern Fetal Neonatal Med 2017; 30(4): 386-96.
       [http://dx.doi.org/10.3109/14767058.2016.1174210] [PMID: 27052666]

[80]   Musso D, Rouault E, Teissier A, *et al.* Molecular detection of Zika virus in blood and RNA load determination during the French Polynesian outbreak. J Med Virol 2017; 89(9): 1505-10.
       [http://dx.doi.org/10.1002/jmv.24735] [PMID: 27859375]

[81]   Landry ML, St George K. Laboratory Diagnosis of Zika Virus Infection. Arch Pathol Lab Med 2017; 141(1): 60-7.
       [http://dx.doi.org/10.5858/arpa.2016-0406-SA] [PMID: 27763787]

[82]   Chan PA, Robinette A, Montgomery M, *et al.* Extragenital Infections Caused by Chlamydia trachomatis and Neisseria gonorrhoeae: A Review of the Literature. Infect Dis Obstet Gynecol 2016; 2016: 5758387.
       [http://dx.doi.org/10.1155/2016/5758387] [PMID: 27366021]

[83]   Silasi M, Cardenas I, Kwon JY, Racicot K, Aldo P, Mor G. Viral infections during pregnancy. Am J Reprod Immunol 2015; 73(3): 199-213.
       [http://dx.doi.org/10.1111/aji.12355] [PMID: 25582523]

[84]   Adams Waldorf KM, McAdams RM. Influence of infection during pregnancy on fetal development. Reproduction 2013; 146(5): R151-62.
       [http://dx.doi.org/10.1530/REP-13-0232] [PMID: 23884862]

[85]   Gonococcal Infections. 2015. www.cdc.gov/std/tg2015/gonorrhea.htm

[86]   Centers for Disease Control and Prevention. Sexually transmitted disease surveillance report 2003.Atlanta (GA)7 US Department of Health and Human Services, Centers for Disease Control and Prevention. 2004.

[87]   Howie SE, Horner PJ, Horne AW. Chlamydia trachomatis infection during pregnancy: known unknowns. Discov Med 2011; 12(62): 57-64.
       [PMID: 21794209]

[88]   Andrews WW, Goldenberg RL, Mercer B, *et al.* The Preterm Prediction Study: association of second-

trimester genitourinary chlamydia infection with subsequent spontaneous preterm birth. Am J Obstet Gynecol 2000; 183(3): 662-8.
[http://dx.doi.org/10.1067/mob.2000.106556] [PMID: 10992190]

[89]   Kohl KS, Markowitz LE, Koumans EH. Developments in the screening for *Chlamydia trachomatis*: A review. Obstet Gynecol Clin North Am 2003; 30(4): 637-58.
[http://dx.doi.org/10.1016/S0889-8545(03)00076-7] [PMID: 14719842]

[90]   Brocklehurst P, Rooney G. Interventions for treating genital *Chlamydia trachomatis* infection in pregnancy. Cochrane Database Syst Rev 2000; (2): : CD000054.
[PMID: 10796106]

[91]   Cooper WO, Ray WA, Griffin MR. Prenatal prescription of macrolide antibiotics and infantile hypertrophic pyloric stenosis. Obstet Gynecol 2002; 100(1): 101-6.
[PMID: 12100810]

[92]   Adimora AA. Treatment of uncomplicated genital *Chlamydia trachomatis* infections in adults. Clin Infect Dis 2002; 35 (Suppl. 2): S183-6.
[http://dx.doi.org/10.1086/342105] [PMID: 12353204]

[93]   Magriples U, Copel JA. Can risk factor assessment replace universal screening for gonorrhea and Chlamydia in the third trimester? Am J Perinatol 2001; 18(8): 465-8.
[http://dx.doi.org/10.1055/s-2001-18790] [PMID: 11733863]

[94]   Stamm LV. Syphilis: Re-emergence of an old foe. Microb Cell 2016; 3(9): 363-70.
[http://dx.doi.org/10.15698/mic2016.09.523] [PMID: 28357375]

[95]   Wahab AA, Ali UK, Mohammad M, Md Monoto EM, Rahman MM. Syphilis in pregnancy. Pak J Med Sci 2015; 31(1): 217-9.
[PMID: 25878647]

[96]   Watson-Jones D, Changalucha J, Gumodoka B, *et al.* Syphilis in pregnancy in Tanzania. I. Impact of maternal syphilis on outcome of pregnancy. J Infect Dis 2002; 186(7): 940-7.
[http://dx.doi.org/10.1086/342952] [PMID: 12232834]

[97]   Genc M, Ledger WJ. Syphilis in pregnancy. Sex Transm Infect 2000; 76(2): 73-9.
[http://dx.doi.org/10.1136/sti.76.2.73] [PMID: 10858706]

[98]   Lumbiganon P, Piaggio G, Villar J, *et al.* WHO Antenatal Care Trial Research Group. The epidemiology of syphilis in pregnancy. Int J STD AIDS 2002; 13(7): 486-94.
[http://dx.doi.org/10.1258/09564620260079653] [PMID: 12171669]

[99]   Augenbraun MH. Treatment of syphilis 2001: nonpregnant adults. Clin Infect Dis 2002; 35 (Suppl. 2): S187-90.
[http://dx.doi.org/10.1086/342106] [PMID: 12353205]

[100] Wendel GD Jr, Sheffield JS, Hollier LM, Hill JB, Ramsey PS, Sánchez PJ, *et al.* Treatment of syphilis in pregnancy and prevention of congenital syphilis. Clin Infect Dis 2002; 35 (Suppl. 2): S200-9.
[http://dx.doi.org/10.1086/342108] [PMID: 12353207]

[101] Marai W. Lower genital tract infections among pregnant women: a review. East Afr Med J 2001; 78(11): 581-5.
[http://dx.doi.org/10.4314/eamj.v78i11.8947] [PMID: 12219963]

[102] Mullick S, Watson-Jones D, Beksinska M, Mabey D. Sexually transmitted infections in pregnancy: prevalence, impact on pregnancy outcomes, and approach to treatment in developing countries. Sex Transm Infect 2005; 81(4): 294-302.
[http://dx.doi.org/10.1136/sti.2002.004077] [PMID: 16061534]

CHAPTER 6

Anti-Infective Agents for HIV in Pregnancy

Igor Thiago Queiroz*, **Themis Rocha Souza, Juliana Mendonça Freire, Alexandre Estevam Montenegro Diniz** and **Matheus de Araújo Duda**

Medicine School, Potiguar University, Sen. Salgado Filho Av., 1610, Natal, Rio Grande do Norte, Zip Code 59056-600, Brazil

Abstract: The use of antiretrovirals in pregnant women is mandatory to suppress HIV replication and prevent mother-to-child vertical transmission, and some drugs are available to compound such therapeutic regimens. Infectious disease specialists and obstetricians have to work together with the aim to diminish the teratogenic effects of each drug and to protect the fetus from the virus. Herein, the most popular antiretroviral drugs are discussed, regarding their mechanism of action, adverse events and safety of use in pregnancy.

Keywords: AIDS, Antiretroviral, HIV, Pregnancy, Treatment.

BACKGROUND

Discovered in the early 1980s, Human Immunodeficiency Virus (HIV) is a member of the *Lentivirus* genus, from the *Retroviridae* family. After HIV attachment to the host cell (CD4 receptor and then to CCR5 or CXCR4 co-receptor), the fusion of the viral envelope with the host cell membrane occurs, and the nucleocapsid is internalized. Once inside the host cell, the HIV genome is released and a reverse transcriptase enzyme is used to convert HIV's RNA into DNA, allowing migration of viral DNA to the nucleus of the host cell and integration with the host DNA by integrase enzyme. Later, this integrated DNA is transcribed in messenger RNA which is translated into long-chain polyproteins that are cleaved by proteases, giving rise to viral proteins [1, 2].

HIV is known to attack immune cells (mainly CD4+ T lymphocytes) and to gradually provoke immunodeficiency during natural infection. It is transmitted between human beings through unprotected sexual practices, sharing needles among illicit drug users, transfusion of blood (and also their derivatives), tissue

---

* **Corresponding author Igor Thiago Queiroz:** Medicine School, Potiguar University (UnP), Sen. Salgado Filho Av., 1610, Natal, Rio Grande do Norte, Zip Code 59056-600, Brazil; Tel: +55843215 1273; E-mail: igor.queiroz@unp.br

Ricardo Ney Cobucci (Ed.)

and organ transplants, occupationally, and vertically during pregnancy, delivery and breastfeeding [2].

Diagnosing HIV infection is mandatory in vulnerable people that exhibit certain risky behaviors, as cited above regarding transmission, mainly if they show some signs and symptoms that demonstrate failure in the immune system or if they have established the acquired immunodeficiency syndrome (AIDS). Serologic and molecular methods such as Enzyme-Linked Immunosorbent Assay (EIA), Indirect Immunofluorescence (IF), Western Blot, Polymerase Chain Reaction, and Rapid tests are available to diagnose HIV in public and private health [2].

The World Health Organization (WHO) recommends that every pregnant woman should be tested for HIV infection as early as possible in each pregnancy and should repeat the HIV test in the third trimester of pregnancy or during childbirth due to the high risk of contraction during this period [3].

Usually, initiating treatment is generally a non-emergency intervention and is something that has to be agreed upon between the doctors and their patients, and the concerns are: the willingness and readiness to promptly initiate antiretroviral therapy (ART); the drugs to be chosen (as well as dosage, scheduling, likely benefits, possible adverse effects); and the required long-term follow-up visits that come after. The WHO guidelines recommend ART initiation as soon as the diagnosis of HIV infection is established, regardless of CD4+ T lymphocyte count or disease stage and some studies show certain benefits with this practice [3]. Concerning pregnant women, ART initiation has to be accelerated, and the drug regimen requires attention to rapid viral suppression (preventing vertical transmission), avoiding teratogenic adverse effects in the fetus, and has to be continued throughout the mother's life after delivery [4, 5].

The first cases of HIV infection in children were reported in June 1983 and immediately following this discovery researchers began to try to understand the mode of transmission and how to avoid it [6]. Two years later, in December 1985, the US Public Health Service published the first recommendations to prevent mother-to-child transmission of HIV [7]. However, these were not followed until 1994 when there was a historical landmark for prevention of mother-to-child transmission of HIV as the Department of US Health and Human Services issued treatment guidelines for pregnant women living with HIV, recommending the use of Zidovudine for pregnant women [8]. Over the years, new therapy combinations have been developed and studied to decrease the rate of mother-to-child transmission of HIV, to lower toxicity and costs, and to enhance its benefits. The use of ARV during pregnancy, injectable AZT during labor, the cesarean delivery when high viral loads are detected in pregnant women, as well as administration of postpartum AZT in newborns exposed to HIV, and non-breastfeeding are some of the measures recommended for the success of vertical non-transmission.

A large number of antiretrovirals are available for the treatment of HIV infected people, especially pregnant women. As an example, the WHO currently recommends as the first-line drugs for pregnant women the combination of tenofovir disoproxil fumarate (TDF) 300 mg, lamivudine (3TC) 300 mg or emtricitabine (FTC) 300 mg, and Dolutegravir 50 mg taken orally once a day, based on their convenience, simplicity, safety and effectiveness. Another therapeutic regimen accepted is based on the combination of TDF 300 mg, 3TC/FTC 300 mg and Efavirenz 600 mg [9].

In light of this, it is vital to include this often-marginalized group of pregnant women in antiretroviral clinical research. Hence, the main drugs and drug combinations, resistance mechanisms, and teratogenicity are of fundamental importance to ascertain proper management of this group of patients, contributing to a lower rate of vertical transmission, providing the mother with protection against the possible effects of AIDS, and generating a lower cost in public health.

From this point on, each drug will be discussed separately by class, focusing on the treatment of HIV-infected pregnant women.

ANTIRETROVIRALS FOR HIV INFECTED PREGNANT WOMAN

Treatment of any disease becomes more effective and reliable when it is based on clinical research and scientific evidence. Since there is no difference in HIV infection in pregnant women, the choice of a therapeutic regimen should be based on the analysis of clinical studies published in specialized journals. For example, the ARV registration site for pregnant women (http://www.apregistry.com/) provides valuable and safe information on this subject.

In 1996, at the 11th International AIDS Conference (Vancouver, Canada), a mixture using protease inhibitors known as the drug cocktail was presented, which reduced the HIV reproduction rate by 100 times as compared to antiviral treatment in monotherapy [10].

Thus, the regimen chosen for pregnant women, non-pregnant women, children, and adolescents contains at least three agents. The treatment utilized should be discussed and selected with each patient, so that they are informed of the benefits and risks, durability and tolerability of the medications, and that the best therapeutic adherence can occur [11].

The treatment has to be individualized according to the HIV story of the pregnant woman, in regard to resistance or comorbidities. In general, pregnant women who are already on ART should remain on their regimen unless the levels of the drug used are higher than recommended or there are known adverse effects for the mother, fetus, or newborn. There are different scenarios for choosing a therapeutic regimen for pregnant women including those that have never received any ARV drugs, those that have already had prophylaxis, those that have become pregnant during a previous ARV regimen, or for those that are changing the regimen because it is not well tolerated [11].

The chosen drugs should be evaluated for safety during pregnancy. The drugs are divided into different categories that are listed on the Chemical Hazards emergency medical management website (https://chemm.nlm.nih.gov/pregnancy categories.htm).

NUCLEOS(T)IDE ANALOG REVERSE-TRANSCRIPTASE INHIBITORS (NRTI)

Used primarily as an anticancer drug since 1964, but with a poor response for this purpose, zidovudine was the first NRTI approved in 1987 for use against HIV. Results shown by PACTG 076 were the first major discovery against HIV infection, revealing a 67.5% reduction in vertical transmission [12].

This class is represented by five drugs: Zidovudine (AZT), Abacavir (ABC), Tenofovir Disoproxil Fumarate (TDF), Lamivudine (3TC), and Emtricitabine (FTC). The defining mechanism of action of these drugs is by interfering with HIV reverse transcriptase by competitive inhibition. Such nucleoside analogs have three stages of intracellular phosphorylation for the formation of the nucleoside triphosphate, which is the active drug moiety. Unlike the rest, TDF (a nucleotide analog) has an adenine-based monophosphate component and requires only two phosphorylation steps to form the active moiety [11].

Clinical trials presented by American guidelines showed no evidence of teratogenicity in any of these five NRTI, and they demonstrated a high rate of transduction from the placenta to the fetus. Preferable combinations of this class in pregnant women are 3TC alone, ABC+3TC, or TDF+FTC [11].

Class Representatives

Zidovudine or Azidotimidine (ZDV or AZT)

Mechanism of Action and Resistance

A synthetic thymidine analog which is potent *in vitro* activity against other retroviruses, AZT/ZDV terminates the elongation of DNA after intracellular phosphorylation and also by diminishing the amount of thymidine triphosphate due to competitive inhibition of cellular thymidine kinase enzyme. Some Thymidine Analog Mutations (TAMs) which have the capacity of cross-resistance to other thymidine analogs (such as stavudine) occur mainly when AZT/ZDV is used in monotherapy [13].

Untoward Effects

Most frequently, zidovudine may cause hematologic toxicity, including granulocytopenia, anemia, and headache. It can cause myopathy, myositis, and liver toxicity, but this is unusual [4]. Furthermore, symptoms, such as fatigue, malaise, myalgia, nausea and insomnia, are common adverse events. Erythrocyte macrocytosis is seen in almost everyone who takes this medication but is not associated with anemia. Other effects due to chronic use are nail hyperpigmentation, myopathy, hepatic toxicity, and lactic acidosis [13, 14].

Use in Pregnancy

Due to its wide exposure, zidovudine is approved for the prevention of mother-to-child transmission of HIV infection. The administration of oral ZDV in rats during pregnancy did not show embryotoxicity when doses 23 times higher than those used in humans were administered. As for studies in humans, both PACTG076 and PACT219/219C have also shown no evidence of teratogenicity [11].

Tenofovir Disoproxil Fumarate (TDF)

Mechanism of Action and Resistance

The only nucleotide analog used against HIV infection, TDF is marketed as a disoproxil prodrug, augmenting its bioavailability (absorption and cellular penetration). Mutation in only one codon (K65R) is responsible for TDF resistance, which can be partially restored by M184V mutation [13].

Untoward Effects

Even though it is not toxic to human renal tubular cells, *in vitro* TDF can cause rare episodes of acute renal failure and Fanconi's syndrome, so it has to be used with caution in those with preexisting renal disease, and renal function and phosphorus have to be evaluated constantly. Combined use with didanosine (ddI) is contraindicated and due to interactions with drug transporters, combined use with atazanavir, ritonavir or lopinavir/ritonavir has to be checked more frequently [5, 13].

Use in Pregnancy

TDF is approved for use in adults, including pregnant women, mainly in combination with Lamivudine or Emtricitabine. An observational study in Botswana of approximately 11,000 births among women with HIV on ART therapy did not show adverse events at birth, such as stillbirth or neonatal death; on the contrary, the risks were higher in patients who used alternative regimens [15].

Abacavir (ABC)

Mechanism of Action and Resistance

A synthetic carbocyclic purine analog, ABC is the only guanosine analog approved for use in humans. Codon substitutions (K65R, L74V, Y115F, and M184V) are responsible for producing modest resistance, which is augmented when they are combined [16].

Untoward Effects

Fatal hypersensitivity syndrome is the main adverse event of abacavir, it is reported in approximately 2-9% of patients and is associated with the HLA-B*5701 locus. The drug has to be suspended and can never be restarted. Other symptoms are headache, malaise, fever, abdominal pain, cough, dyspnea, and musculoskeletal pain. Large doses of ethanol can increase ABC plasma levels and restrict its elimination [5, 13].

Use in Pregnancy

ABC is approved for use in children up to three months old and in adults, including pregnant women, mainly in combination with lamivudine or zidovudine [6]. Studies with rats have shown no evidence of increased malformation in fetuses when doses of abacavir up to 700mg/Kg are used. As for human studies, the SMARTT (Surveillance Monitoring for ART Toxicities) and the French

Perinatal Study also showed no evidence of fetal malformation from exposure to ABC in the first trimester of pregnancy [17, 18].

Lamivudine (3TC)

Mechanism of Action and Resistance

3TC is a cytidine analog reverse transcriptase inhibitor which is phosphorylated after entering into the cells by passive diffusion. A single amino-acid substitution (M184V or M184I) is responsible for lamivudine resistance, high-level cross-resistance to emtricitabine, and a lesser degree resistance to abacavir, thus maintaining or restoring susceptibility to zidovudine and tenofovir [19].

Untoward Effects

As it has a low affinity to human DNA polymerase, revealing low toxicity to the host, lamivudine shows fewer toxic effects and few adverse events [6]. Most frequently, 3TC causes headaches, fatigue, nausea, diarrhea, skin rash, and abdominal pain. However, in more severe cases, it can cause pancreatitis (primarily seen in children with advanced HIV infection receiving multiple other medications), peripheral neuropathy, decreased neutrophil count, and increased liver enzymes [20].

Use in Pregnancy

3TC is approved for use in children up to three months old and adults, including pregnant women, mainly in combination with TDF or AZT [9]. No evidence of teratogenicity was shown in studies with rats and rabbits that had plasma concentrations of 3TC 35 times higher than plasma in humans [19]. According to the antiretroviral pregnancy registry, there were no significant differences in fetal formation in those 11,000 pregnant women exposed to 3TC when compared to the US population of the Metropolitan Atlanta Congenital Defects Program [11].

Emtricitabine (FTC)

Mechanism of Action and Resistance

FTC is a cytidine analog that shares many characteristics with 3TC, including its mechanism of action and resistance [20].

Untoward Effects

Hyperpigmentation of skin (in sun-exposed areas) can occur with prolonged use of FTC [20].

Use in Pregnancy

FTC is approved for use in adults, including pregnant women, mainly in combination with TDF or AZT [6]. In a randomized study in which three groups were compared (placebo, TDF, and TDF+FTC) no differences in congenital abnormalities were observed between those groups [21]. Another large study (PHACS/SMARTT) also did not report teratogenicity when using this drug in pregnancy [17].

NON-NUCLEOSIDE ANALOG REVERSE-TRANSCRIPTASE INHIBITORS (NNRTI)

In 1996, the FDA approved Nevirapine (the first known NNRTI) for the treatment of HIV-1 infection. Since then, researchers have carried out studies on pregnant women to compare its accuracy in relation to AZT, which was confirmed by the HIVNET012 study in Uganda [22]. However, they perceived a certain resistant mutation (K103N) in those women who received Nevirapine for the prevention of vertically transmitted HIV [23]. From then on, it was decided that drug combinations should be used for the prevention of mother-to-child transmission (PMTCT), thus avoiding the rise of mutation rates in HIV infected patients.

Acting through the same mechanism of action of the NRTI by blocking the elongation of proviral DNA, NNRTI were discovered by iterative screening and are composed of five drugs: Efavirenz (EFV), Nevirapine (NVP), Etravirine (ETV), Rilpivirine (RPV), and Doravirine (DOR). As a non-competitive inhibitor, NNRTI binds to a hydrophobic pocket of reverse transcriptase of HIV, which is far from the active site, inducing a conformational change in the structure of the enzyme. They do not require intracellular phosphorylation to perform their activity and do not interact with host cell DNA polymerases. All of them have hepatic metabolism and may cause potential toxicity to the liver [13]. NNRTI based regimens have demonstrated virologic potency and durability. However, a therapeutic scheme containing efavirenz or rilpivirine has a high prevalence of primary resistance in naive patients with a low genetic barrier. Therefore, resistance testing should be performed before initiating therapy in pregnant women [13].

Class Representatives

Efavirenz (EFV)

Mechanism of Resistance and Action

As mentioned above EFV acts on inhibiting the reverse transcriptase by binding directly to the enzyme. A single mutation (K103N) is responsible for decreasing susceptibility by up to 100 times and there is some cross-resistance to nevirapine and delavirdine, contraindicating the use of these drugs in patients that have failed their first therapeutic regimen previously [13].

Untoward Effects

Nearly half of patients experience some side effects related to the central nervous system (dizziness, dysphoria, disturbing or vivid dreams, impaired concentration or insomnia) or psychiatric ones (depression, psychosis, hallucinations and mania), but with a low rate of discontinuation because these are resolved in a few weeks. Rash can occur in a quarter of adults in the first weeks of treatment [11]. Also, there is a detected high risk of suicidal or self-injury behaviors among those who use EFV, as well as an elevation in LDL-c and triglycerides [3].

Use in Pregnancy

The FDA recommends health care providers avoid administering this drug during the first gestational trimester, because there are some studies that show the teratogenicity of EFV [11]. A study conducted on monkeys going through the first gestational trimester found some malformations in the central nervous system and cleft palate in 3 out of 20 newborn monkeys [24]. In addition, an increase in microcephaly rate in HIV-exposure was found in a recent report from the Pediatric HIV/AIDS Cohort Study (PHACS) [25].

Nevirapine (NVP)

Mechanism of Action and Resistance

The mechanism of action is similar to that described for EFV, as both are from the same class. A single mutation in 103 or 181 codons is responsible for resistance and a two-fold decrease in its action, with a high level of resistance and clinical treatment failure, which is extended to EFV and delavirdine [13].

Untoward Effects

Most frequently, NVP may cause skin rash (some severe and life-threatening, including Stevens-Johnson syndrome), sedative effect, headache, diarrhea, and nausea. It abnormally causes elevated liver enzymes and, rarely, hepatitis [3].

Use in Pregnancy

According to data gathered by the antiretroviral pregnancy registry, there was no increase in cardiovascular defects or genitourinary system in those infants exposed to NVP, and this drug is approved for use in adults, infants and children up to 15 days of life, being allowed to be used in pregnancy to prevent mother-to-child transmission [13].

Etravirine (ETV)

Mechanism of Action and Resistance

Having a similar mechanism of action, ETV has a high genetic mutation barrier compared to EFV, NVP or Delavirdine [14]. New studies have shown that a mutation at position E138 is considered as a Resistance mechanism for ETV [26].

Untoward Effects

Rash is the only adverse event present with ETV, occurring in the first weeks of use. As an inducer of CYP3A4 and glucuronosyltransferases, it can induce some drug interactions [13].

Use in Pregnancy

Etravirine is classified by the Food and Drug Administration as Category B for pregnancy. There is not sufficient data to adequately assess the risk of major birth defects, miscarriage or adverse maternal or fetal outcomes [27].

Rilpivirine (RPV)

Mechanism of Action and Resistance

RPV shows a low barrier of resistance, similar to EFV, and there are some ART-naive patients that show primary resistance to this drug. In patients treated with RPV, the presence of mutations may confer cross-resistance to other NNRTIs [28].

Untoward Effects

Depression, headache, skin rash, and QT prolongation are some adverse events of RPV use [29].

Use in Pregnancy

There is no difference in the overall risk of birth defects for RPV compared with the background treatment rate for major birth defects of 2.7% in the Metropolitan Atlanta Congenital Defects Program (MACDP) reference population, and the rate of miscarriage is not reported in the Antiretroviral Pregnancy Registry (APR) [29].

Doravirine (DOR)

Mechanism of Action and Resistance

DOR has an *in vitro* resistance profile that is distinct from other NNRTI and retains activity against viruses containing the most frequently transmitted NNRTI mutations. Thus, the prevalence of resistance is lower in comparison to other NNRTI [30].

Untoward Effects

Being generally well tolerated DOR has fewer adverse events than EFV or RPV. According to the FDA, some of the adverse events are nausea, dizziness, headache, fatigue, diarrhea, abdominal pain, and abnormal dreams [31].

Use in Pregnancy

No adequate human data are available to establish whether or not DOR poses a risk to pregnancy outcomes and the mothers are instructed not to breastfeed if they are receiving it [31]. In animal studies, no toxicological effects were observed in the embryo/fetus of rats and rabbits and in pre/post-natal rats when doses 9 times higher were used in humans [31].

PROTEASE INHIBITORS (PI)

In 1995, Saquinavir (SQV) was the first protease inhibitor approved for use in HIV treatment associated with NRTI. Currently, this class is represented by three main drugs: Atazanavir (ATV), Darunavir (DRV), and Ritonavir (RTV) [5].

Protease inhibitors are peptide-like chemicals that competitively inhibit the action of the virus aspartyl protease. These drugs prevent proteolytic cleavage of HIV gag and pol precursor polypeptides that include the essential structural (p17, p24, p9, and p7) and enzymatic (reverse transcriptase, protease, and integrase) components of the virus. This prevents the metamorphosis of HIV virus particles into their mature infectious form [13, 32].

Class Representatives

Atazanavir (ATV)

Mechanism of Action and Resistance

ATV is an azapeptide protease inhibitor that is active against both HIV-1 and HIV-2 [33]. It binds reversibly to the active site of HIV protease, preventing the polypeptide processing and subsequent viral maturation. The viral replication, in the presence of Atazanavir, leads to the selection of drug resistance [34]. The primary ATV resistance mutation confers about a 9-fold decreased susceptibility [6]. Sensitivity to atazanavir is affected by various primary and secondary mutations that accumulate in patients who have failed other HIV protease inhibitors, with high-level resistance more likely if five or more additional mutations are present [33].

Untoward Effects

ATV frequently causes indirect hyperbilirubinemia, although this is mainly a cosmetic side effect and is not associated with hepatotoxicity. Other side effects reported with ATV include diarrhea and nausea, mainly during the first few weeks of therapy [14], PR interval prolongation, especially in patients who have underlying conduction defects or who are on concomitant medications that can cause PR prolongation, hyperglycemia, fat maldistribution, cholelithiasis, nephrolithiasis, renal insufficiency, serum transaminase elevations, hyperlipidemia (especially with RTV boosting), and skin rash [3, 29].

Use in Pregnancy

There is a fast reduction of viral load, with low placental transfer to fetus, no evidence of human teratogenicity, effect of in utero ATV exposure on infant indirect bilirubin levels is unclear, and nonpathological elevations of neonatal hyperbilirubinemia have been observed in some, but not all, clinical trials to date, but monitoring bilirubin levels in the newborn is recommended [35, 36]. A French cohort study found no birth defects in those children exposed to the drug in the first trimester of pregnancy [37].

Darunavir (DRV)

Mechanism of Action and Resistance

DRV has bimodal activity against HIV-1 protease, enzymatic inhibition and protease dimerization inhibition, and has an extremely high genetic barrier against the development of drug resistance [38].

Untoward Effects

DRV contains a sulfa moiety and rash has been reported in up to 10% of recipients. Although causality is not firmly established, darunavir has been associated with episodes of hepatotoxicity [3, 13, 35]. Darunavir/Ritonavir is associated with increases in plasma triglycerides and cholesterol, although the magnitude of the increase is lower than that seen with Lopinavir/Ritonavir [39].

Use in Pregnancy

According to data gathered by the antiretroviral pregnancy registry, there is no evidence of an increase in teratogenicity in those children exposed to DRV in the first gestational trimester. Furthermore, in animal studies, embryotoxicity was not found in those rats that received doses of DRV 3 times higher than those recommended for human use [40]. Monitoring hepatic function is necessary, especially in the first few months of use and if there is pre-existing liver disease [5, 35].

Ritonavir (RTV)

Mechanism of Action and Resistance

The mechanism of action of RTV is similar to ATV. Viral particles are produced in the presence of RTV but are not infectious [13]. Ritonavir is mostly used as a pharmacokinetic enhancer (CYP3A4 inhibitor), and the low doses used for this purpose are not known to induce ritonavir resistance mutations [34].

Untoward Effects

The major side effects of ritonavir are gastrointestinal (GI) and include dose-dependent nausea, vomiting, diarrhea, anorexia, abdominal pain, and taste perversion. GI toxicity may be reduced if the drug is taken with meals. Peripheral and perioral paresthesias can occur at the therapeutic dose of 600 mg twice daily. These side effects generally subside within a few weeks of starting therapy. Ritonavir also causes dose-dependent elevations in serum total cholesterol and triglycerides, as well as other signs of lipodystrophy, and it could increase the long-term risk of atherosclerosis in some patients [13].

Use in Pregnancy

Although there is low placental transfer to fetus and no evidence of human teratogenicity, the oral solution contains 43% of alcohol RTV and is therefore not recommended during pregnancy, because there is no known safe level of alcohol exposure during pregnancy [11].

INTEGRASE INHIBITORS (INI)

Over the years, the evolution of HIV studies has brought an improvement in the quality of ARV, promoting more potent, safer drugs, with fewer side effects and providing a better quality of life for HIV patients. This class of drugs is currently used as first-line medication in several therapeutic regimens. Raltegravir and Dolutegravir are the two main examples of this class. STARTMARK was the first study that proved the superiority of Raltegravir compared to Efavirenz in naïve patients starting treatment [41]. Following Dolutegravir approval in 2013 by the FDA, several studies have shown its effectiveness and safety in relation to other drugs [42]. Chromosomal integration is a defining characteristic of retrovirus life cycles and allows viral DNA to remain in the host cell nucleus for a prolonged period of inactivity or latency. Because human DNA is not known to undergo excision and reintegration, this is an excellent target for antiviral intervention. It prevents the formation of covalent bonds between host and viral DNA [13].

Class Representatives

Dolutegravir (DTG)

Mechanism of Action and Resistance

The mechanism of action is similar to the integrase inhibitor class. Regarding the mechanism of resistance, DTG has shown, within its class, a differentiated profile, since the resistant strain selection has not been found so far in first-line regimens [39].

Untoward Effects

DTG is generally well tolerated. The most commonly reported adverse reactions of moderate-to-severe intensity were insomnia and headache. Case series of neuropsychiatric adverse events (sleep disturbances, depression, anxiety, suicidal ideation) associated with the initiation of DTG and RAL have been reported [29]. Hepatotoxicity and hypersensitivity reactions have also been reported [3].

Use in Pregnancy

The World Health Organization recommends the use of DTG associated with two other NRTI as the first-line treatment for all groups of patients, including pregnant and non-pregnant women [9]. Despite the reports of four cases of neural tube malformation in Botswane, new studies have shown the effectiveness and safety of DTG in pregnant women and found no association of DTG with neural tube malformation. Currently, it is the preferred drug for use throughout pregnancy and an alternative drug for women who are trying to conceive. The use of folic acid 400 mg per day is recommended for those women who want to conceive or who are pregnant [11].

Raltegravir (RAL)

Mechanism of Action and Resistance

RAL blocks the catalytic activity of the HIV-encoded integrase, thus preventing the integration of virus DNA into the host chromosome. RAL produces potent activity against both HIV-1 and HIV-2 and retains activity against viruses that have become resistant to antiretroviral agents of other classes because of its unique mechanism of action. The two major RAL resistance pathways involve primary mutations in the integrase gene [13].

Untoward Effects

RAL use has been associated with creatine kinase elevations, myositis and rhabdomyolysis. Rare cases of severe skin reactions and systemic hypersensitivity reactions in patients who received RAL have been reported during post-marketing surveillance. Neuropsychiatric adverse events (*e.g.*, insomnia, headache, depression, and suicidal ideation) have been reported in people taking integrase strand transfer inhibitors [29]. Hepatotoxicity, severe skin rash and hypersensitivity reactions have also been reported [3, 35].

Use in Pregnancy

Although there is high placental transfer to the fetus, there is no evidence of human teratogenicity as shown in IMPAACT P1026s, in P1097, in PANNA studies, and in other case reports [11]. There is a report of markedly elevated liver transaminases with RAL use in late pregnancy. Severe, potentially life-threatening, and fatal skin and hypersensitivity reactions have been reported in non-pregnant adults [11].

ENTRY AND FUSION INHIBITORS

The first steps of the HIV infection life cycle are from the fusion and entry of viral particles into human cells. These two classes are intended to prevent these stages of the viral cycle. The main example of Entry Inhibitors (Mavirock) act by inhibiting the interaction of the chemokine co-receptor CCR5 with HIV gp120.

The FDA-approved fusion inhibitor (Enfurtivide) was the first approved ARV that acts extracellularly by inhibiting viral entry. Enfuvirtide (T20) and Maraviroc (MVC) are not recommended for initial ART in pregnancy. Its uses are recommended for rescue therapy in patients multi-experienced with various class drugs and who have not had viral suppression with the first line [11].

Class Representatives

Maraviroc (MRV)

<u>*Mechanism of Action and Resistance*</u>

Maraviroc is a chemokine receptor antagonist and binds to the host cell CCR5 receptor to block binding of viral gp120. It blocks the binding of the HIV outer envelope protein gp120 to the CCR5 chemokine receptor. It is active only against CCR5-tropic strains of HIV and has no activity against viruses that are CXCR4-tropic or that have dual-tropism [43]. MRV retains activity against viruses that have become resistant to antiretroviral agents of other classes because of its unique mechanism of action. HIV can develop resistance to this drug through two distinct pathways. A patient starting maraviroc therapy with HIV that has predominantly CCR5-tropism may experience a shift in tropism to CXCR4 or dual/mixed-tropism predominance. This is especially likely in patients harboring low-level but undetected CXCR4 or dual/mixed-tropic virus prior to initiation of maraviroc. Alternatively, HIV can retain its CCR5-tropism but gain resistance to the drug through specific mutations in the V3 loop of gp120 that allows virus binding in the presence of inhibitor [13, 43].

<u>*Untoward Effects*</u>

Maraviroc is generally well tolerated, with little significant toxicity. Abdominal pain, cough, dizziness, musculoskeletal symptoms, pyrexia, rash, upper respiratory tract infections, hepatotoxicity, which may be preceded by severe rash or other signs of systemic allergic reactions, and orthostatic hypotension, especially in patients with severe renal insufficiency, have been reported [13, 29].

<u>*Use in Pregnancy*</u>

Although there is moderate placental transfer to the fetus, there is no evidence of teratogenicity in rats or rabbits, and there is insufficient data to assess for teratogenicity in humans [9]. MVC requires a test of tropism (CCR5 or CXCR4) prior to its use. There are few reports of use during pregnancy [5, 11].

Enfuvirtide (T20)

Mechanism of Action

Enfuvirtide inhibits fusion of the viral and cell membranes mediated by gp41 and CD4 interactions. This drug retains activity against viruses that have become resistant to antiretroviral agents of other classes because of its unique mechanism of action. HIV can develop resistance to this drug through specific mutations in the enfuvirtide-binding domain of gp41 [44].

Untoward Effects

Local injection site reactions (*e.g.*, pain, erythema, induration, nodules and cysts, pruritus, and ecchymosis) occur in almost 100% of patients; increased incidence of bacterial pneumonia; hypersensitivity reactions occur in <1% of patients, and the symptoms may include rash, fever, nausea, vomiting, chills, rigors, hypotension, or elevated serum transaminases [11].

Use in Pregnancy

Enfuvirtide is classified by the Food and Drug Administration as Category B for pregnancy. There is minimal to low placental transfer to fetus and there is no data on human teratogenicity. However, because there are no studies on the safe use of this medication during pregnancy, it is not recommended for use in pregnant women. *In vitro* and *in vivo* studies suggest that enfuvirtide does not readily cross the human placenta. Minimal placental passage of enfuvirtide was reported in published studies that included a total of eight peripartum patients and their neonates [45].

CONSIDERATIONS ABOUT USE OF ANTIRETROVIRALS INTRAPARTUM AND AFTER DELIVERY

The administration of intrapartum zidovudine depends on the HIV viral load of the mother near the delivery and should be used regardless of the presence of resistance. It is indicated when HIV-RNA > 1000 copies/mL, HIV RNA at unknown levels or poor adherence to ART is suspected; on the other hand, if HIV-RNA is consistently < 1000 copies/mL the use of zidovudine intrapartum is not specifically recommended [46]. Since 1993, Protocol 076 has been responsible for recommending the use of AZT in labor, demonstrating a reduction from 25.5% to 8.3% in those newborns exposed to HIV [12].

Despite the initiation of ART in all pregnant women during the gestational period in order to diminish mother-to-child transmission of HIV and for their own clinical benefit, all infants born to HIV-infected mothers should receive post-exposure antiretroviral prophylaxis to prevent exposure to HIV during delivery and for four to six weeks of life (preferably within 6 to 12 hours of life. The recommended scheme depends on the infant's risk of infection as determined by timing of maternal infection (previous to or during pregnancy) and their use of ART, and type of infant feeding – breastfeeding or receiving replacement feeding [47]. Thus, for those mothers who have had a low risk of transmission, that is, those who had viral suppression <50 copies during the entire pregnancy, AZT should be administered for 4 weeks in those children. In the case of Higher Risk of Perinatal HIV Transmission, the therapy used is ZDV, 3TC, and NVP (treatment dose) or ZDV, 3TC, and RAL for up to 6 weeks. In general, the use of ART is considered safe in infants [11] (Table **1**).

Table 1. HIV post-exposure prophylaxis in newborns from HIV-infected women. Adapted from Panel on Treatment of Pregnant Women with HIV Infection and Prevention of Perinatal Transmission. Recommendations for Use of Antiretroviral Drugs in Transmission in the United States. Accessed 2020 July 6th . Available from https://aidsinfo.nih.gov/contentfiles/lvguidelines/PerinatalGL.pdf.

Level of Perinatal HIV Transmission Risk	Definition	Neonatal ARV Management
Low Risk of Perinatal HIV Transmission	For mothers who were medicated with ART during pregnancy and that had sustained viral suppression (the definition is set according to a confirmed HIV RNA level), and there is no concern about adherence.	ZDV for 28 days or four weeks.
Higher Risk of Perinatal HIV Transmission	For mothers who were neither medicated with ARV antepartum nor intrapartum drugs. For mothers who were medicated only with intrapartum ARV drugs. For mothers who were medicated with both antepartum and intrapartum ARV drugs but who presented evident viral loads close to delivery, especially when they had vaginal delivery. Mothers with acute or primary HIV infection during pregnancy or breastfeeding (in which case, it is advisable that the mother interrupt breastfeeding)	Possible HIV therapy that can use ZDV, 3TC, and NVP (treatment dose) or ZDV, 3TC, and RAL administered from the moment of birth until 42 days or six weeks.

(Table 1) contd.....

Presumed Newborn HIV Exposure	Mothers with HIV diagnoses not yet confirmed but who have tested positive at least once at delivery or postpartum or whose newborns have tested positive for HIV antibody.	ARV administration such as that described above is for newborns with a higher risk transmission of perinatal HIV. ARV drugs for newborns should be interrupted right away if complementary testing confirms that the mother does not test positive for HIV.
Newborn with HIV infection	Positive newborn HIV virologic test/NAT.	Treatment doses with a three-drug ARV regimen.

CONCLUSION

Antiretroviral use in pregnant women is one of the various ways of preventing mother-to-child transmission of HIV and these drugs should be carefully studied to guarantee safe use in pregnant women, avoiding adverse events in gestation, whether for the woman or the fetus. The best regimen to be followed worldwide depends on the region and on the country (respecting each one's national guidelines), thus a three-drug association seems to be the best option.

CONSENT FOR PUBLICATION

Not applicable.

CONFLICT OF INTEREST

The authors declare no conflict of interest, financial or otherwise.

ACKNOWLEDGEMENTS

Declared none.

REFERENCES

[1]   The HIV Life Cycle Understanding HIV/AIDS [Internet]. AIDSinfo. 2020 [cited 9th July 2020]. Available from: https://aidsinfo.nih.gov/understanding-hiv-aids/fact-sheets/19/73/the-hiv-life-cycle

[2]   Sax PE. The natural history and clinical features of HIV infection in adults and adolescents. UpToDate [Accessed on January 24th, 2019] 2019.https://www.uptodate.com/contents/the-natural-history--nd-clinical-features-of-hiv-infection-in-adults-and-adolescents

[3]   Consolidated guidelines on HIV testing services. 1st ed. Geneva: World Health Organization 2015. Available: apps.who.int/iris/bitstream/handle/10665/179870/9789241508926_eng.pdf?sequence=1

[4]   Consolidated Guidelines on the Use of Antiretroviral Drugs for Treating and Preventing HIV Infection: Recommendations for a Public Health App roach. 2nd edition. Geneva: World Health Organization 2016. Available: www.ncbi.nlm.nih.gov/books/NBK374294/

[5]   Brasil Ministério da Saúde Secretaria de Vigilância em Saúde Departamento de Vigilância, Prevenção e Controle das Infecções Sexualmente Transmissíveis, do HIV/Aids e das Hepatites Virais Protocolo

Clínico e Diretrizes Terapêuticas para Prevenção da Transmissão Vertical do HIV, da Sífilis e das Hepatites Virais / Ministério da Saúde, Secretaria de Vigilância em Saúde, Departamento de Vigilância, Prevenção e Controle das Infecções Sexualmente Transmissíveis, do HIV/Aids e das Hepatites Virais. Brasília: Ministério da Saúde 2018; p. 248.

[6] Wayne EK, Gould Michele, M Flynn Patrick. HIV/AIDS and Substance Abuse. In: Miller PM, Eds. Interventions for addiction. 3rd ed. London: Academic Press 2013; pp. 235-42.

[7] Centers for Disease Control (CDC). Recommendations for Assisting in the Prevention of Perinatal Transmission of Human T-lymphotropic Virus Type III/lymphadenopathy-associated Virus and Acquired Immunodeficiency SyndromeMMWR1985 34: 32-721.

[8] Current Trends Recommendations for Assisting in the Prevention of Perinatal Transmission of Human T-Lymphotropic VirusType III/Lymphadenopathy-Associated Virus and AcquiredImmunodeficiency Syndrome [Internet]. Cdc.gov. 2020 [cited 7th July 2020]. Available from: https://www.cdc.gov/mmwr/preview/mmwrhtml/00033122.htm

[9] Update of recommendations on first- and second-line antiretroviral regimens Geneva, Switzerland: World Health Organization; 2019 (WHO/CDS/HIV/1915) Licence: CC BY-NC-SA 30 IGO 2019.

[10] Yount L. A to Z of biologists. 1st ed., New York, NY: Facts on File 2003.

[11] Panel on Treatment of Pregnant Women with HIV Infection and Prevention of Perinatal Transmission. Recommendations for Use of Antiretroviral Drugs in Transmission in the United States http://aidsinfo.nih.gov/contentfiles/lvguidelines/PerinatalGL.pdf

[12] Connor EM, Sperling RS, Gelber R, *et al.* Reduction of maternal-infant transmission of human immunodeficiency virus type 1 with zidovudine treatment. Pediatric AIDS Clinical Trials Group Protocol 076 Study Group. N Engl J Med 1994; 331(18): 1173-80. [http://dx.doi.org/10.1056/NEJM199411033311801] [PMID: 7935654]

[13] Goodman LS, Brunton LL, Chabner B, Knollmann BC. Goodman & Gilman's the pharmacological basis of therapeutics. 12th ed., New York: McGraw-Hill Medical Pub 2011.

[14] Goodman LS, Gilman A, Brunton LL, Lazo JS, Parker KL. Goodman & Gilman's the pharmacological basis of therapeutics. 11th ed., New York: McGraw-Hill Medical Pub 2006.

[15] Zash R, Rough K, Jacobson DL, *et al.* Effect of gestational age at tenofovir-emtricitabine-efavirenz initiation on adverse birth outcomes in Botswana. J Pediatric Infect Dis Soc 2018; 7(3): e148-51.https://www.ncbi.nlm.nih. gov/pubmed/29688554 [http://dx.doi.org/10.1093/jpids/piy006] [PMID: 29688554]

[16] Abacavir [package insert] Food and Drug Administration 2018. Available at: https://www.accessdata.fda.gov/drugsatfda_docs/label/2018/020977s033s034,020978s036s037lbl.pdf

[17] Williams PL, Crain MJ, Yildirim C, *et al.* Pediatric HIV/AIDS Cohort Study. Congenital anomalies and in utero antiretroviral exposure in human immunodeficiency virus-exposed uninfected infants. JAMA Pediatr 2015; 169(1): 48-55. http://www.ncbi. nlm.nih.gov/pubmed/25383770 [http://dx.doi.org/10.1001/jamapediatrics.2014.1889] [PMID: 25383770]

[18] Sibiude J, Le Chenadec J, Bonnet D, *et al.* In utero exposure to zidovudine and heart anomalies in the ANRS French perinatal cohort and the nested PRIMEVA randomized trial. Clin Infect Dis 2015; 61(2): 270-80. http://www.ncbi.nlm. nih.gov/pubmed/25838291 [http://dx.doi.org/10.1093/cid/civ260]

[19] Lamivudine [package insert] Food and Drug Administration 2018. Available at: https://www.accessdata.fda.gov/drugsatfda_docs/label/2018/020564s038,020596s037lbl.pdf

[20] Emtricitabine [package insert] Food and Drug Administration 2018. Available at: https://www.accessdata.fda.gov/ drugsatfda_docs/label/2018/021896s026lbl.pdf

[21] Mugo NR, Hong T, Celum C, *et al.* Partners PrEP Study Team. Pregnancy incidence and outcomes among women receiving preexposure prophylaxis for HIV prevention: a randomized clinical trial.

JAMA 2014; 312(4): 362-71. http://www.ncbi.nlm.nih.gov/pubmed/25038355
[http://dx.doi.org/10.1001/jama.2014.8735] [PMID: 25038355]

[22]   Guay LA, Musoke P, Fleming T, *et al*. Intrapartum and neonatal single-dose nevirapine compared with zidovudine for prevention of mother-to-child transmission of HIV-1 in Kampala, Uganda: HIVNET 012 randomised trial. Lancet 1999; 354(9181): 795-802.
[http://dx.doi.org/10.1016/S0140-6736(99)80008-7] [PMID: 10485720]

[23]   Jackson JB, Becker-Pergola G, Guay LA, *et al*. Identification of the K103N resistance mutation in Ugandan women receiving nevirapine to prevent HIV-1 vertical transmission. AIDS 2000; 14(11): F111-5.
[http://dx.doi.org/10.1097/00002030-200007280-00001] [PMID: 10983633]

[24]   Nightingale SL. From the food and drug administration. JAMA 1998; 280(17): 1472.
[http://dx.doi.org/10.1001/jama.280.17.1472-JFD80010-3-1] [PMID: 9809716]

[25]   Williams PL, Yildirim C, Chadwick EG, *et al*. Surveillance monitoring for ART toxicities (SMARTT) study of the pediatric HIV/AIDS cohort study. Association of maternal antiretroviral use with microcephaly in children who are HIV-exposed but uninfected (SMARTT): a prospective cohort study. Lancet HIV 2020; 7(1): e49-58. https://www.ncbi.nlm.nih.gov/pubmed/31740351
[http://dx.doi.org/10.1016/S2352-3018(19)30340-6] [PMID: 31740351]

[26]   Xu HT, Colby-Germinario SP, Asahchop EL, *et al*. Effect of mutations at position E138 in HIV-1 reverse transcriptase and their interactions with the M184I mutation on defining patterns of resistance to nonnucleoside reverse transcriptase inhibitors rilpivirine and etravirine. Antimicrob Agents Chemother 2013; 57(7): 3100-9.
[http://dx.doi.org/10.1128/AAC.00348-13] [PMID: 23612196]

[27]   Etravirine. AIDSinfo [internet]; (2019). [Accessed on January 24th , 2019]. Available in: https://aidsinfo.nih.gov/drugs/398/etravirine/16/professional

[28]   Rilpivirine. AIDSinfo [internet]. [Accessed on January 24th, 2019]. Available in 2019.https://aidsinfo.nih.gov/drugs/426/rilpivirine/19/professional

[29]   Panel on Antiretroviral Guidelines for Adults and Adolescents. Guidelines for the Use of Antiretroviral Agents in Adults and Adolescents Living with HIV http://aidsinfo.nih.gov/contentfiles/lvguidelines/AdultandAdolescentGL.pdf

[30]   Soulie C, Santoro MM, Charpentier C, *et al*. Rare occurrence of doravirine resistance-associated mutations in HIV-1-infected treatment-naive patients. J Antimicrob Chemother 2018.
[https://doi.org/10.1093/jac/dky464].
[PMID: 30476106]

[31]   Doravirine [package insert] Food and Drug Administration 2019. Available at: https://www.accessdata.fda.gov/ drugsatfda_docs/label/2019/210806s003lbl.pdf

[32]   Flexner C. HIV-protease inhibitors. N Engl J Med 1998; 338(18): 1281-92.
[http://dx.doi.org/10.1056/NEJM199804303381808] [PMID: 9562584]

[33]   Croom KF, Dhillon S, Keam SJ. Atazanavir: a review of its use in the management of HIV-1 infection. Drugs 2009; 69(8): 1107-40.
[http://dx.doi.org/10.2165/00003495-200969080-00009] [PMID: 19496633]

[34]   Goodman LS, Gilman A, Brunton LL, Lazo JS, Parker KL. Goodman & Gilman's the pharmacological basis of therapeutics. 11th ed., New York: McGraw-Hill Medical Pub 2006.

[35]   Brasil Ministério da Saúde Secretaria de Vigilância em Saúde Departamento de Vigilância, Prevenção e Controle das Infecções Sexualmente Transmissíveis, do HIV/Aids e das Hepatites Virais Protocolo Clínico e Diretrizes Terapêuticas para Manejo da Infecção pelo HIV em Adultos / Ministério da Saúde, Secretaria de Vigilância em Saúde, Departamento de Vigilância, Prevenção e Controle das Infecções Sexualmente Transmissíveis, do HIV/Aids e das Hepatites Virais. Brasília: Ministério da Saúde 2018; p. 412.

[36]   Atazanavir   [packageinsert]   Food   andDrugAdministration   2018.   Available   at: https://www.accessdata.fda.gov/drugsatfda_docs/label/2018/021567s042,206352s007lbl.pdf

[37]   Sibiude J, Mandelbrot L, Blanche S, *et al.* Association between prenatal exposure to antiretroviral therapy and birth defects: an analysis of the French perinatal cohort study (ANRS CO1/CO11). PLoS Med 2014; 11(4)e1001635http://www.ncbi.nlm.nih.gov/pubmed/24781315 [http://dx.doi.org/10.1371/journal.pmed.1001635] [PMID: 24781315]

[38]   Aoki M, Das D, Hayashi H, *et al.* Mechanism of Darunavir (DRV)'s High Genetic Barrier to HIV-1 Resistance. A Key V32I Substitution in Protease Rarely Occurs, but Once It Occurs, It Predisposes HIV-1 To Develop DRV Resistance. mBio 2018; 9(2): 17.e02425 Published 2018 Mar 6

[39]   McKeage K, Perry CM, Keam SJ. Darunavir: a review of its use in the management of HIV infection in adults. Drugs 2009; 69(4): 477-503. [http://dx.doi.org/10.2165/00003495-200969040-00007] [PMID: 19323590]

[40]   Darunavir   [package   insert]   Food   and   Drug   Administration   2019.   Available   at: https://www.accessdata.fda.gov/drugsatfda_docs/label/2019/021976s054,202895s025lbl.pdf

[41]   Lennox JL, Dejesus E, Berger DS, *et al.* Raltegravir *versus* Efavirenz regimens in treatment-naive HIV-1-infected patients: 96-week efficacy, durability, subgroup, safety, and metabolic analyses. J Acquir Immune Defic Syndr 2010; 55(1): 39-48. [published correction appears in J Acquir Immune DeficSyndr. 2011 Dec 1;58(4):e120]. [http://dx.doi.org/10.1097/QAI.0b013e3181da1287] [PMID: 20404738]

[42]   Nunes EP. Dolutegravir *versus* raltegravir em pacientes em falha à terapia antirretroviral estudo Sailing.   Braz   J   Infect   Dis   2:   16-23.   Available   from: http://www.bjid.org.br/en-pdf-X2177511716525050

[43]   MacArthur RD, Novak RM. Reviews of anti-infective agents: maraviroc: the first of a new class of antiretroviral agents. Clin Infect Dis 2008; 47(2): 236-41. [http://dx.doi.org/10.1086/589289] [PMID: 18532888]

[44]   Dando TM, Perry CM. Enfuvirtide. Drugs 2003; 63(24): 2755-66. [http://dx.doi.org/10.2165/00003495-200363240-00005] [PMID: 14664654]

[45]   Enfuvirtide   [package   insert]   Food   and   Drug   Administration   2015.   Available   at: http://www.accessdata.fda.gov/ drugsatfda_docs/label/2015/021481s030lbl.pdf

[46]   Hughes B, Cu-Uvin S. Antiretroviral and intrapartum management of pregnant HIV-infected women and their infants in resource-rich settings UpToDate [Internet] [Accessed on January 24th, 2019]. Available   in   https://www.uptodate.com/contents/antiretroviral-and-intrapartum-managemen--of-pregnant-hiv-infected-women-and-their-infants-in-resource-rich-settings

[47]   Flynn PM, Abrams EJ, Fowler MG. Prevention of mother-to-child HIV transmission in resource-limited   settings   2019.   https://www.uptodate.com/contents/prevention-of-mother-to-chil--hiv-transmission-in-resource-limited-settings

CHAPTER 7

Anti-Infective Agents for Vulvovaginal Infections in Pregnancy

Iaponira da Silva Figueiredo Vidal, Ana Paula Costa, Ana Katherine Gonçalves and **Maria da Conceição de Mesquita Cornetta**[*]

Federal University of Rio Grande do Norte, Nilo Peçanha Av., 259, Natal, Brazil

Abstract: This chapter discusses genital changes in the gestational period and their influences in the vaginal microbiome. Using the latest scientific evidence, the most common genital infections will be shown, as well as the best methods of diagnosis and the use of antibacterials agents in the gestational period, with their recommended strength.

Keywords: Bacterial vaginosis, Genital vulvovaginal candidiasis, Pregnancy, Trichomonas infections, Vulvovaginitis, Vulvovaginal infections.

BACKGROUND

The main concern about the association of vulvovaginal infections and pregnancy is whether they carry any consequences to the mother or the fetus. During pregnancy, hormone elevation of estrogen can determine physiological genital changes, such as increased lactic acid, to defend the vagina from infectious diseases that can reach the uterine cavity and impair pregnancy and the fetus. The increase in PH is a result of glycogen metabolism following apoptosis of superficial cells of the vaginal epithelium during estrogen-induced epithelial maturation, which is increased during pregnancy [1].

Genital Changes During Pregnancy

The pregnancy period means important hormonal changes in the maternal body and it is known that the microbiome both affects and is affected by the hormones that influence bacterial growth [2]. Vaginal content increases during pregnancy and is manifested by a white discharge with a pH range from 3.5 to 6 [1]. This vaginal acid environment is enhanced by the presence of lactobacilli which contributes to its growth [3]. Estrogen present during pregnancy accelerates

---

[*] **Corresponding author Maria da Conceição Cornetta:** Federal University of Rio Grande do Norte, Nilo Peçanha Av., 259, Natal, Brazil; Tel: +558432155969; E-mail: mcornetta@hotmail.com

maturation of the squamous epithelium until desquamated cells release their glycogen into the vaginal environment, which is metabolized into lactic acid and causes a decrease in local pH, this can then prevent the bacterial from ascending through the vagina. This is the initial knowledge that explains the vaginal changes during pregnancy, that is until several authors started to bring to the scientific community many more explanations, such as the description of the microbiome and its changes during pregnancy, although further research is needed to clarify some gaps [1, 3, 4].

Agaard [3] reported the discovery, using special techniques, that the vaginal microbiome during pregnancy was enriched in *Lactobacillus iners, Lactobacillus crispatus, Lactobacillus jensenii,* and *Lactobacillus johnsonii,* this is possibly because of the increased estrogen. Knowledge about the microbiome is important and related to the mode of delivery, be it a cesarean section or vaginal delivery, which interferes with the microbiome of the newborn and is capable of influencing the composition of his/her immune system [3]. Vaginal infection causes premature rupture of the membranes that can determine premature birth and neonatal deaths because it leads to the production of cytokines that can bring on labor. The poor pregnancy outcome can be determined from *gardnerella, mycoplasma* and *anaerobes* [5].

One of the main consequences of infection in pregnancy is prematurity, a result of the premature rupture of the membranes, responsible for many fetal and neonatal deaths in developing countries. These infections develop from the vagina and trigger the production of cytokines that cause uterine contractions and begin labor [6].

Currently, knowledge about the bacterial population of the genital tract shows the interaction with certain diseases and the diversity of the vaginal microbiome is different in each woman. This may result in some obstetric complications, such as preterm delivery [4].

The presence of *Lactobacillus* in the vagina is very important to prevent the ascendence of the bacterial and can limit their growth by decreasing the pH. In general, a low educational level and certain occupations are considered risk factors for vaginitis, but, in particular, the vaginitis-related bacteria may be a cause of increased perinatal mortality [7]. Romero [8] observed that the pregnant vaginal tract composition and stability are different from the non-pregnant one, with a predominance of *Lactobacillus ssp* in the microbial community. A cohort study [9] showed that there is an association of decreased richness, diversity and less stability in the genital microbiome with preterm birth. A recent study [10] suggests that despite *Lactobacillus* vaginal diversity, the presence of BV-associated bacteria may be associated with early preterm birth, although further studies are recommended taking into consideration the immunological factors. On the other hand, it is possible to find reports showing the relationship of bacterial taxa associated with dysbiosis in the expression of proinflammatory cytokines expression and preterm birth. In fact, certain data, such as clinical and genetic factors, metabolic and immunologic biomarkers, when associated, may be considered useful in defining the preterm birth risk [11].

All these modifications can be associated with vulvovaginitis and poor pregnancy results. The three most important and common genital infectious diseases during pregnancy are Bacterial Vaginosis, Trichomoniasis and Candidiasis, which will be described below. At the end of the description, there will be a Table **1** with a list of medicines that are most commonly used for the treatment of these diseases.

Bacterial vaginosis (BV), a very common vaginal dysbiosis in pregnancy, and is one of the most common causes of vaginal discharge in women of reproductive age. The prevalence of these infections varies by race, ranging from 5 to 15% in caucasian females and up to 55% in black women. The occurrence of candidiasis, on the other hand, affects 29 to 49% of the female population and affects approximately 50% of women in Germany [12, 13].

BACTERIAL VAGINOSIS

Bacterial vaginosis (BV) is the most common cause of abnormal discharge, although a lot of the time it is asymptomatic. In typical cases, the vaginal discharge has a fishy odor [14]. This clinical syndrome results from the replacement of the common H_2O_2-producing *Lactobacillus* species in the vagina with high concentrations of anaerobic bacteria (*e.g., Prevotella* spp and *Mobiluncus* spp), as well as with *Gardnerella vaginalis*, and Mycoplasma hominis [15].

The pathophysiology of the microbial alteration is not fully understood, particularly in pregnancy [16]. BV during pregnancy may be associated with adverse pregnancy outcomes, including premature rupture of the membranes, preterm labor, preterm birth, chorioamnionitis, post-abortion endometritis, and postpartum endometritis [17].

The diagnosis can be made clinically in the presence of three of these four criteria: homogeneous discharge, vaginal pH higher than 4.5, positive amine test, and the presence of clue cells in the bacterioscopic examination. However, just the presence of fetid odor and clue cells are sufficient for the diagnosis, because of the importance of these two criteria. Diagnosis can also be made by using just a gram-stained vaginal bacterioscopy, or by identifying certain morphological types of bacteria involved in this infection, such as *Gardnerella vaginalis* and

Mobiluncus spp, and by the decrease or absence of *Lactobacillus* [18].

The treatment of BV during gestation is recommended, using oral metronidazole 500 mg BID x 7 days or 250 mg TID x 7 days, and the alternative treatment is Tinidazole 2 grams orally a day x 2 days or Tinidazole 1 gram orally x 5 days [19]. Treatment of the sexual partner is not recommended because it is not a Sexually Transmitted Disease. Topical and short-term treatments have been shown to be much less effective than long-term oral treatments (five to seven days). The time of treatment is also fundamental, and it should be instituted as early as possible in prenatal care in order to obtain the best results [20]. When it is administered before 20 weeks of gestation and in women with abnormal vaginal flora, the treatment has better results, although much more information is necessary to support screening and treatment can reduce premature birth (before 37 weeks of pregnancy), as well as perinatal morbidity and mortality [21]. Screening and treatment of asymptomatic pregnant women remain controversial, although there is a benefit for those with previous preterm birth [14].

TRICHOMONAS VAGINALIS

The *Trichomonas vaginalis* is a flagellated protozoan parasite of the human genital tract and the cause of the most prevalent curable sexually transmitted disease globally, with an estimated 276.4 million cases per year, worldwide [22]. The primary symptom of trichomoniasis in women is vaginal discharge, but approximately half of all women are asymptomatic. Trichomonas infection in pregnancy has been associated with preterm premature rupture of membranes, preterm delivery, and low birthweight in infants [23].

Diagnosis of trichomoniasis in female patients is frequently carried out microscopically, with the examination of a "wet mount" of vaginal or cervical exudates for motile parasites. This method is very simple to carry out, fast and cost-effective, when compared with alternative diagnostic options, including culture or molecular methods. Despite these advantages, microscopic evaluation is not considered the optimal detection method, due to the low sensitivity offered by this technique [24]. The culture of *T. vaginalis* from clinical samples has long been regarded as the gold standard for the diagnosis of this organism. Serological methods for diagnosing from vaginal secretions have been developed, but are rarely used clinically. Both commercial, and "in house" PCR based assays are available and provide a more sensitive form of testing than the traditional methods of wet-mount microscopy and culture [25, 26].

The standard treatment for *T. vaginalis* infection is a single 2 g oral dose of metronidazole or tinidazole and the alternative treatment is metronidazole 500 mg BID x 7 days [19]. A significant cause of treatment failure in metronidazole therapy is resistance to the drug [27]. A significant cause of treatment failure in metronidazole therapy is resistance to the drug [27].

CANDIDIASIS

The etiologic agent of vulvovaginal candidiasis (VVC) is typically *Candida albicans*, but infections with other Candida spp can occur. Vaginal candidiasis is the most common cause of infectious vulvovaginitis during pregnancy. Clinically, it may manifest through white or curd-like discharge accompanied by vulvovaginal pruritus and eventually dysuria, vulvar burning, and excoriation. Despite this, this typical picture is not always present, commonly causing a confusing diagnosis during pregnancy [28].

Children born of normal birth from mothers with candidiasis can be colonized with *Candida albicans* and develop oral candidiasis, compromising breastfeeding. These babies can also develop diaper dermatitis at some point in their lives, being more frequent in the 2nd to 4th weeks. For this reason, the treatment of asymptomatic infection is recommended in the final weeks of pregnancy in Germany [29]. Although colonization of the vagina and cervix with Candida is generally characterized by benign commensalism, under certain conditions, when maternal immunity is severely compromised (*e.g.*, AIDS), uterine fungal infection can occur upwards. Intrauterine infection by Candida is very rare but extremely severe to the fetus [30].

The diagnosis of VVC is often made clinically by the presence of typical symptoms and signs, supplemented by the identification of yeast on a wet mount or using culture [31]. Clotrimazol was the most frequently prescribed CVV treatment in Germany [13].

Treatment of vaginal infections in pregnancy should be done as early as possible, as they can cause miscarriages and premature birth. There is no evidence that the use of Metronidazole in the first trimester of pregnancy as well as during breastfeeding is related to teratogenic effects or neonatal complications. [32, 12]. Symptomatic women should be treated at diagnosis to avoid complications in pregnancy. The use of metronidazole seems to be safe at any stage of pregnancy as well as during lactation, only causing a change in taste. manufacturers recommend discontinuing breastfeeding for 12 to 24 hours after single-dose metronidazole use. The use of Tinidazole, in turn, has shown adverse events with its use in animals and there is no evidence of its safe use in human pregnancy [12] Clindamycin use in the first half of pregnancy to treat vaginal infections prevents late miscarriage, premature birth and low birth weight [33].

For the treatment of vulvovaginal candidiasis, there is a consensus on the vaginal use of medications. A study conducted in Denmark using oral Fluconazole showed an increased risk of miscarriage and fetal death, others have reported the occurrence of tetralogy of Fallot [12, 34]. Treatment of candidiasis in pregnancy should preferably be performed with topical imidazole, with no difference in superiority between them. The cure rate reaches 90% with seven-day treatment [35].

Table 1. Antimicrobial Agents for the Treatment of Vaginal Infections in Pregnancy.

Vaginal Infection	Best Treatment Recommended	Method of Administration
BV/ TV	Metronidazol	2000 mg/single dose
BV/ TV	Metronidazol	0.75% vaginal cream/7 days
BV/ TV	Metronidazol	2% vaginal cream/7 days
Candidosis	Clotrimazol	1% vaginal cream/7-14 days
Candidosis	Nistatine	10,000 U vaginal cream/14 days
Candidosis	Butoconazol	vaginal cream/ 3 days
Candidosis	Miconazol	vaginal cream/ 7 days
Candidosis	Tioconazol	vaginal cream/ 3 days
Candidosis	Terconazol	0.4g vaginal cream/ 7 days
Candidosis	Terconazol	0.8g vaginal cream/ 3 days

Source: McDonald, HM *et al.*, 2001; Sherrad, J *et al.*, 2018.

CONCLUSION

The current best recommendations from the European guidelines for the management of the three genital infections in pregnant women are:

For TV, metronidazole. Strength of recommendation: Grade 1, quality of evidence: Grade A. For BV, clindamycin. Strength of recommendation: Grade 2, quality of evidence: Grade C, and for Candida, topical azole preparations. Strength of recommendation: Grade 1, quality of evidence: Grade B.

CONSENT FOR PUBLICATION

Not applicable.

CONFLICT OF INTEREST

The authors declare no conflict of interest, financial or otherwise.

ACKNOWLEDGEMENTS

Declared none.

REFERENCES

[1]   Amabebe E, Anumba DOC. The vaginal microenvironment: The physiologic role of *Lactobacilli*. Front Med (Lausanne) 2018; 5: 181.
[http://dx.doi.org/10.3389/fmed.2018.00181] [PMID: 29951482]

[2]   Nuriel-Ohayon M, Neuman H, Koren O. Microbial changes during pregnancy birth, and infancy. Front Microbiol 2016; 7: 1031.

[3]   Aagaard K, Riehle K, Ma J, *et al.* A metagenomic approach to characterization of the vaginal microbiome signature in pregnancy. PLoS One 2012; 7(6): : e36466.
[http://dx.doi.org/10.1371/journal.pone.0036466] [PMID: 22719832]

[4]   Prince AL, Chu DM, Seferovic MD, Antony KM, Ma J, Aagaard KM. The perinatal microbiome and pregnancy: moving beyond the vaginal microbiome. Cold Spring Harb Perspect Med 2015; 5(6): a023051.
[http://dx.doi.org/10.1101/cshperspect.a023051] [PMID: 25775922]

[5]   Aroutcheva AA, Simões JA, Faro S. Antimicrobial protein produced by vaginal *Lactobacillus acidophilus* that inhibits *Gardnerella vaginalis*. Infect Dis Obstet Gynecol 2001; 9(1): 33-9.
[http://dx.doi.org/10.1155/S1064744901000060] [PMID: 11368257]

[6]   Goldenberg R L, Hauth J C, Andrews W W. Intrauterine infection and preterm delivery. N Engl J Med 2000; 342(20): 1500-5.

[7]   Xu F, Du X, Xie L. Vaginitis in pregnancy is related to adverse perinatal outcome. Pak J Med Sci 2015; 31(3): 582-6.
[PMID: 26150848]

[8]   Romero R, Hassan SS, Gajer P, *et al.* The composition and stability of the vaginal microbiota of normal pregnant women is different from that of non-pregnant women. Microbiome 2014; 2(1): 4.
[http://dx.doi.org/10.1186/2049-2618-2-4] [PMID: 24484853]

[9]   Stout MJ, Zhou Y, Wylie KM, Tarr PI, Macones GA, Tuuli MG. Early pregnancy vaginal microbiome trends and preterm birth. Am J Obstet Gynecol 2017; 217(3): 356.e1-356.e18.
[http://dx.doi.org/10.1016/j.ajog.2017.05.030] [PMID: 28549981]

[10]   Tabatabaei N, Eren AM, Barreiro LB, *et al.* Vaginal microbiome in early pregnancy and subsequent risk of spontaneous preterm birth: a case-control study. BJOG 2019; 126(3): 349-58.
[http://dx.doi.org/10.1111/1471-0528.15299] [PMID: 29791775]

[11]   Fettweis JM, Serrano MG, Brooks JP, *et al.* The vaginal microbiome and preterm birth. Nat Med 2019; 25(6): 1012-21.
[http://dx.doi.org/10.1038/s41591-019-0450-2] [PMID: 31142849]

[12]   Sherrard J, Wilson J, Donders G, Mendling W, Jensen JS. European (IUSTI/WHO) guideline on the management of vaginal discharge. Int J STD AIDS 2018; 29(13): 1258-72.
[http://dx.doi.org/10.1177/0956462418785451] [PMID: 30049258]

[13]   Jacob L, John M, Kalder M, Kostev K. Prevalence of vulvovaginal candidiasis in gynecological practices in Germany: A retrospective study of 954,186 patients. Curr Med Mycol 2018; 4(1): 6-11.
[http://dx.doi.org/10.18502/cmm.4.1.27] [PMID: 30186987]

[14]   Sobel JD. Bacterial vaginosis: Treatment. In: Robert L. Barbieri, Ed. Up To Date Wayne State University School of Medicine Up To Date , 2019 https://www.uptodate.com/contents/bacterial-vaginosis-treatment [Accessed february 21,2019];

[15]   Yudin MH. Bacterial vaginosis in pregnancy: diagnosis, screening, and management. Clin Perinatol

2005; 32(3): 617-27.
[http://dx.doi.org/10.1016/j.clp.2005.05.007] [PMID: 16085023]

[16]   Nelson DB, Macones G. Bacterial vaginosis in pregnancy: current findings and future directions. Epidemiol Rev 2002; 24(2): 102-8.
[http://dx.doi.org/10.1093/epirev/mxf008] [PMID: 12762086]

[17]   Thurman AR, Doncel GF. Innate immunity and inflammatory response to *Trichomonas vaginalis* and bacterial vaginosis: relationship to HIV acquisition. Am J Reprod Immunol 2011; 65(2): 89-98.
[http://dx.doi.org/10.1111/j.1600-0897.2010.00902.x] [PMID: 20678168]

[18]   Rao SR, Pindi KG, Rani U, Sasikala G, Kawle V. Diagnosis of bacterial vaginosis: Amsel's criteria vs. Nugent's scoring. Sch J Appl Med Sci 2016; 4(6C): 2027-31.
[http://dx.doi.org/10.21276/sjams.2016.4.6.32]

[19]   Workowski KA, Bolan GA. Sexually transmitted diseases treatment guidelines, 2015. MMWR Recomm Rep 2015; 64(RR-03): 1-137.
[PMID: 26042815]

[20]   Brocklehurst P, Gordon A, Heatley E, Milan SJ. Antibiotics for treating bacterial vaginosis in pregnancy. Cochrane Database Syst Rev 2013; (1):
[http://dx.doi.org/10.1002/14651858.CD000262.pub4]

[21]   Thinkhamrop J. Antibiotics for treating bacterial vaginosis in pregnancy: RHL commentary (last revised: 4 July 2007). The WHO Reproductive Health Library. Geneva: World Health Organization 2007.

[22]   Global incidence and prevalence of selected curable sexually transmitted infections – 2008. Geneva, Switzerland: World Health Organisation 2012.

[23]   Bachmann LH, Hobbs MM, Seña AC, *et al.* *Trichomonas vaginalis* genital infections: progress and challenges. Clin Infect Dis 2011; 53(S160) (Suppl. 3): S160-72.
[http://dx.doi.org/10.1093/cid/cir705] [PMID: 22080269]

[24]   Bosserman EA, Helms DJ, Mosure DJ, Secor WE, Workowski KA. Utility of antimicrobial susceptibility testing in *Trichomonas vaginalis*-infected women with clinical treatment failure. Sex Transm Dis 2011; 38(10): 983-7.
[http://dx.doi.org/10.1097/OLQ.0b013e318224db39] [PMID: 21934577]

[25]   Garber GE. The laboratory diagnosis of *Trichomonas vaginalis*. Can J Infect Dis Med Microbiol 2005; 16(1): 35-8.
[http://dx.doi.org/10.1155/2005/373920] [PMID: 18159526]

[26]   Patil MJ, Nagamoti JM, Metgud SC. Diagnosis of *Trichomonas vaginalis* from vaginal specimens by wet mount microscopy, in pouch TV culture system, and PCR. J Glob Infect Dis 2012; 4(1): 22-5.
[http://dx.doi.org/10.4103/0974-777X.93756] [PMID: 22529623]

[27]   Muzny CA, Schwebke JR. The clinical spectrum of *Trichomonas vaginalis* infection and challenges to management. Sex Transm Infect 2013; 89(6): 423-5.
[http://dx.doi.org/10.1136/sextrans-2012-050893] [PMID: 23543252]

[28]   Akinbiyi AA, Watson R, Feyi-Waboso P. Prevalence of *Candida albicans* and bacterial vaginosis in Arch Gynecol Obstet. 2008; 278(5): 463-6.

[29]   Mendling W, Spitzbart H. Antimykotische Therapie der vaginalen Hefepilz-Kolonisation von Schwangeren zur Verhütung von Kandidamykosen beim Neugeborenen. AMWF 2008. Guideline 015/042 (S1).

[30]   Mayer FL, Wilson D, Hube B. *Candida albicans* pathogenicity mechanisms. Virulence 2013; 4(2): 119-28.
[http://dx.doi.org/10.4161/viru.22913] [PMID: 23302789]

[31]   Cassone A, Sobel JD. Experimental models of vaginal candidiasis and their relevance to human

candidiasis. Infect Immun 2016; 84(5): 1255-61.
[http://dx.doi.org/10.1128/IAI.01544-15] [PMID: 26883592]

[32]   McDonald HM, Brocklehurst P, Gordon A. Antibiotics for treating bacterial vaginosis in pregnancy. Cochrane Database Syst Rev 2007; (1): : CD000262.
[http://dx.doi.org/10.1002/14651858.CD000262.pub3] [PMID: 17253447]

[33]   Lamont RF, Keelan JA, Larsson PG, Jørgensen JS. The treatment of bacterial vaginosis in pregnancy with clindamycin to reduce the risk of infection-related preterm birth: a response to the Danish Society of Obstetrics and Gynecology guideline group's clinical recommendations. Acta Obstet Gynecol Scand 2017; 96(2): 139-43.
[http://dx.doi.org/10.1111/aogs.13065] [PMID: 27874978]

[34]   Mølgaard-Nielsen D, Svanström H, Melbye M, Hviid A, Pasternak B. Association between use of oral fluconazole during pregnancy and risk of spontaneous abortion and stillbirth. JAMA 2016; 315(1): 58-67.
[http://dx.doi.org/10.1001/jama.2015.17844] [PMID: 26746458]

[35]   Saporiti AM, Gómez D, Levalle S, *et al.* Vaginal candidiasis: etiology and sensitivity profile to antifungal agents in clinical use. Rev Argent Microbiol 2001; 33(4): 217-22.
[PMID: 11833253]

CHAPTER 8

Anti-Infective Agents for Toxoplasmosis in Pregnancy

Igor Thiago Queiroz[1,2,*] and **Carolina A. D. Santos**[2,3,*]

[1] *Hospital Giselda Trigueiro, Natal, Rio Grande do Norte, Brazil*

[2] *Hospital Giselda Trigueiro, Natal - RN, 59037-170, Brazil*

[2] *Instituto Santos Dumont, Macaíba - RN, 59280-000, Brazil*

Abstract: Toxoplasmosis is a global parasitic disease that can be transmitted from mother-to-child when the infection is acquired for the first time during pregnancy. Clinical manifestations of congenital disease include retinochoroiditis, cerebral calcifications, and hydrocephalus. Prenatal testing for toxoplasmosis is routinely offered in many countries so that infected mothers can be treated with antibiotics to reduce the risk of mother-to-child transmission. The diagnosis of toxoplasmosis during pregnancy is complicated because determining whether infection occurred prior to conception or during pregnancy is critical, besides the fact that false-positive tests are common and that there is lack of standardization among these tests. If maternal infection is confirmed before 18 weeks of gestation and the fetus is not yet infected the use of spyramicin is recommended to prevent mother-to-child transmission, as this drug has a high concentration in the placenta and has no teratogenic effects. If infection is presumed or confirmed in the fetus, the treatment should be switched to pyrimethamine, sulfadiazine and folinic acid (PSF) until the end of the gestational period to prevent further damage to the newborn. When maternal infection is confirmed after 18 weeks of gestation, the use of PSF is required, and should be used until delivery. However, these drugs can present some adverse effects, such as paresthesia, pruritus, urticaria, diarrhea, nausea, and vomiting for spiramycin, and arrhythmia, erythema multiforme, pancytopenia, hematuria, and eosinophilic pneumonitis for pyrimethamine. There is an urgent need for having safer drugs on hand that are a suitable chemotherapy or prophylaxis for children and pregnant women, and further studies are needed to address this.

Keywords: Folinic Acid, Pregnancy, Pyrimethamine, Spiramycin, Sulfadiazine, Toxoplasmosis, Treatment.

* **Corresponding authors Igor Thiago Queiroz & Carolina Araújo Damasio Santos:** Hospital Giselda Trigueiro, Natal - RN, 59037-170, Brazil; Tel: +558432327911; E-mails: igor.queiroz@unp.br and damasiocarolina@hotmail.com

Ricardo Ney Cobucci (Ed.)

INTRODUCTION

Toxoplasmosis is a parasitic infection and a worldwide health problem, it is acquired by the ingestion of *Toxoplasma gondii* oocysts excreted by cats which contaminates water or soil, or by eating tissue cysts that remain viable in undercooked meat of infected animals (*e.g.*, pigs, lambs, goats), but that can only be reliably detected by seroconversion (the change from negative to positive *Toxoplasma* specific antibodies). The prevalence varies among adult individuals depending on the studied population and on the age of the individuals [1].

Mother-to-child transmission of the parasite can occur when infection is acquired for the first time during pregnancy. When the parasites are transmitted from the mother to the fetus, the result is congenital toxoplasmosis [1]. Clinical manifestations of congenital disease include retinochoroiditis, cerebral calcifications, hydrocephalus, mental retardation, and even death [2].

The infection in pregnancy is usually asymptomatic and can be detected by serological testing. Prenatal testing for toxoplasmosis is routinely offered in many European countries so that infected mothers can be treated with antibiotics to reduce the risk of mother-to-child transmission and, if fetal infection has occurred, to reduce impairment in the child [3].

The frequency of congenital toxoplasmosis increases with increasing gestational age for maternal infection, but the regularity of severe sequelae in infected offspring is greater when infection occurs early in pregnancy [1]. Overall, vertical transmission occurs in about 25% of pregnancies [2].

In Brazil, seroprevalence varies between 42% and 90% of the population, depending on different regions [4]. A study on pregnant women from primary care clinics from the North Region of Brazil, demonstrated a prevalence of 5.33% of maternal acute infection, and from a study of 487 patients 63.03% had chronic infection. What is more, vertical transmission was confirmed in 28% of the newborns [5]. In a retrospective cohort of pregnant women with acute toxoplasmosis infection from a reference center in Southern Brazil between 2006 and 2016, the fetal rate of congenital toxoplasmosis was 9.2% [4].

This article aims to review the treatments performed on pregnant women glabally and to discuss the options, recommendations and the best therapeutic approach for toxoplasmosis in pregnant women.

SCREENING AND DIAGNOSIS

As maternal infection is usually asymptomatic, serological tests for *Toxoplasma*-specific immunoglobulin M (IgM) and IgG are used to identify infected women during pregnancy at prenatal consultations [6]. IgM antibodies can be detected approximately 14 days after acquisition of toxoplasma infection and decline to undetectable levels after several months. IgG antibodies are detectable 14 days after the first positive IgM test and persist indefinitely [1].

In Brazil, the Ministry of Health recommends universal screening (IgM and IgG) at the first prenatal visit. If the tests are negative, the tests should be performed again every 3 months. If the IgM is negative and the IgG is positive, no supplemental screening is recommended. If the IgM is positive and IgG is negative, another test should be performed in 3 weeks. If the IgG test remains negative, it is a false-positive result and there is no need for treatment. If the IgG is positive, the seroconversion is documented, and treatment is recommended. For women with positive IgM and IgG at the initial screening, an avidity test must be obtained before 16 weeks to establish whether the positive IgM and IgG antibodies reflect recent or chronic infection [7]. High IgG avidity suggests chronic infection (more than four months old) and no treatment is needed in this scenario; low avidity is not diagnostic of recent infection, as low IgG avidity can persist for years [8]. For women who are initially screened at the first trimester and have positive IgM and IgG, the probability that infection occurred after conception is 1 to 3 percent, depending on the test used [6], and it is generally agreed that treatment should also be started.

The diagnosis of toxoplasmosis in asymptomatic pregnant women in which screening is positive is complicated because determining whether infection occurred prior to conception or during pregnancy is critical, and, moreover, false-positive tests are common. What is more, the lack of standardization of the tests can confuse the diagnosis. So, we recommend that toxoplasmosis testing has to be executed by an experienced reference laboratory.

A long-term study followed a large group of women who acquired *Toxoplasma* infection during pregnancy to determine the median and variability of the duration of positive *Toxoplasma*-IgM results. These IgM antibodies were detected for a median of 12.8 months by an immunosorbent agglutination assay and a median of 10.4 months by immunofluorescence test. In 9.1% of women the IgM-positive results lasted longer than 2 years. There were no significant differences in the duration of IgM between women who gave birth to an infected child compared to uninfected child, nor between women treated with pyrimethamine–sulfonamide or spiramycin [6].

Variability in the duration of the IgM response limits its usefulness for predicting the timing of infection in pregnant women, so the decision to offer therapy to reduce the risk of mother to child transmission of *T. gondii* should not be based on a single IgM- and IgG-positive test result alone [6]. If the avidity test is no longer possible, the use of rising IgG titer (two or more from a reference lab) may help the physician estimate the timing of maternal infection and decide on the need for treatment [6].

In pregnant women with acute infection, a monthly obstetric ultrasound should be performed to evaluate fetal findings of congenital toxoplasmosis as these findings can be useful to provide diagnostic and prognostic information. Furthermore, pregnant women with a confirmed or strongly suspected recent infection should be referred to a center specialized in fetal medicine for amniocentesis to obtain a Polymerase Chain Reaction (PCR) for *T. gondii* DNA in amniotic fluid for prenatal diagnosis of fetal infection [9].

MATERNAL (PRENATAL) TREATMENT

Since 1941 sulfonamides have been used as therapeutic agents for treatment of toxoplasmosis. The combined therapy (pyrimethamine and sulfadiazine) was first reported in 1953. Subsequently, spiramycin proved to be effective against tachyzoites in acute infection and pregnant women in order to avoid vertical transmission of toxoplasmosis [10].

No consensus exists about the most effective screening strategy or the best type of treatment [2, 4]. Uncertainty about the benefits of prenatal treatment and concerns about adverse treatment effects and the costs needed to implement prenatal screening have led to diverse policies [4]. Among countries where prenatal screening is performed, recommendations for treatment can differ. In most centers, spiramycin is prescribed immediately after diagnosis of maternal infection and is changed to a pyrimethamine-sulfonamide combination if fetal infection is diagnosed [11]. In Brazil, the Brazilian Ministry of Health recommends serological screening in the first trimester of pregnancy, especially in areas where prevalence is high [7]. While the recommendation of the treatment differs in some centers, the national protocol recommends the use of spiramycin if the diagnosis is before the 30th week of pregnancy, until the end of the pregnancy, and the use of the maternal therapy (pyrimethamine plus sulfadiazine) if the infection occurs after the 30th week of gestation. This drug regimen should be complemented with folinic acid in a way to ameliorate the effects of pyrimethamine, which interferes with folic acid synthesis, as *Toxoplasma* lacks an uptake system for folic acid, although it can be imported by human cells [7].

No randomized trials compared the effects of maternal treatment *versus* no treatment on pregnancy outcomes. In a French survey, most investigators who were surveyed at the time believed that a randomized placebo-controlled clinical trial would be unacceptable, given that spiramycin has been used for this indication in France for more than 30 years [12].

Maternal treatment to reduce the risk of mother-to-child transmission remains controversial. Some of the most robust evidence comes from the Systematic Review on Congenital Toxoplasmosis (SYROCOT), a 2007 systematic review and individual patient meta-analysis data of 20 European cohort studies, from which data of 1438 women was extracted and universal screening for toxoplasmosis in pregnancy was performed. The authors analyzed the effects of timing and type of prenatal treatment on mother-to-child transmission of infection and clinical manifestations before one year of age. Prenatal regimens included spiramycin alone, spiramycin followed by pyrimethamine-sulfonamide, and pyrimethamine-sulfonamide alone. The study found weak evidence that treatment started within 3 weeks of seroconversion reduced mother-to-child transmission compared with treatment started after 8 or more weeks. Gestational age at seroconversion was strongly associated with mother-to-child transmission and with the risk of intracranial lesions, but only marginally with eye lesions. No evidence was found that prenatal treatment significantly reduced the risk of clinical manifestations in infected live born infants. The study could not distinguish whether the reduction in transmission was a real benefit of the treatment or a bias since women were less likely to be treated after a long delay in seroconversion or shortly before delivery unless they had sonographic signs of fetal infection [13].

Observational studies have reported a reduction in mother-to-child transmission after national prenatal maternal screening, fetal diagnosis, and prenatal/postnatal treatment programs were initiated [14]. However, significant differences between treated and untreated women, and the fact that severely affected fetuses that would have died in utero survived as a result of prenatal treatment, could be confounding factors in the impact of treatment on those observed.

Furthermore, there is evidence of a reduction in serious neurological sequelae or postnatal death in children with congenital toxoplasmosis whose mothers were treated during pregnancy. In a European study of a cohort of 293 infected fetuses of whom two-thirds received prenatal treatment, the prenatal treatment reduced the risk of serious neurological sequelae or death by three-quarters [2].

Mandelbrot *et al.* reported on the findings of the first randomized clinical trial (RCT) ever performed on the treatment of acute toxoplasma infection during pregnancy [15]. The authors compared the efficacy and tolerance of pyrimethamine + sulfadiazine *vs.* spiramycin to reduce placental transmission. One hundred and forty-three women were randomized from November 2010 through January 2014. The results showed that amniocentesis with a positive *Toxoplasma gondii* polymerase chain reaction was 10.4% in the pyrimethamine + sulfadiazine group *vs.* 20.3% in the spiramycin group. Also, cerebral ultrasound anomalies appeared in 0/73 fetuses in the pyrimethamine + sulfadiazine group *vs.* 6/70 in the spiramycin group, enabling the authors to conclude that there was a trend towards lower transmission with the pyrimethamine plus sulfadiazine group, but this did not reach statistical significance, possibly due to a lack of statistical power because enrollment to the study was discontinued [15].

Currently, once the diagnosis of toxoplasmosis is established by serologic methods and the recent acquisition of infection is presumed to be during the first 18 weeks of gestation or near conception, treatment of toxoplasmosis with spiramycin is recommended in an attempt to prevent vertical transmission from mother to fetus. However, if fetal infection is confirmed by PCR in amniotic fluid, treatment with pyrimethamine, sulfadiazine and folinic acid is recommended, even if the pregnant woman has already begun spiramycin use [16]. Moreover, if the fetal ultrasound examination suggests congenital toxoplasmosis, the consensus is to administer pyrimethamine-sulfadiazine plus folinic acid [12].

Spiramycin

Spiramycin (a macrolide antibiotic) has a safety profile, it is not teratogenic, and it can be used at any time during pregnancy (preferably before 14 gestational weeks or near delivery), mainly if the screening of the fetus with obstetric ultrasound and PCR is negative [16]. Thus, according to Montoya *et al.* [16], the dose for maternal toxoplasmosis treatment is: Spiramycin: 1,000 mg (or 3 Million Units), orally, every 8 hours a day.

Pyrimethamine, Sulfadiazine, and Folinic Acid (PSF)

With the ability to reduce the risk and severity of long-term symptoms, these combined drugs are administered in cases of confirmed fetal infection and are avoided in the first trimester of pregnancy because of the teratogenic potential and bone marrow toxicity for both mother and fetus [16, 17]. Pharmacokinetic studies have shown their ability to traverse the blood-brain barrier and protect the fetus against malformations. Thus, due to the potential hemato-, renal-, and hepatotoxicity, laboratory testing is required frequently [16].

According to Maldonado *et al.* [18], the dose recognized for toxoplasmosis treatment in pregnancy is:

1. Pyrimethamine (daraprim):

   a. for the first 2 days – 2 mg/kg per day (100 mg), orally, divided twice a day.

   b. from day 3 to 2 months – 1 mg/kg per day (50 mg), orally, every day; may be used until six months when considered for symptomatic congenital toxoplasmosis.

   c. from that point on – 1 mg/kg per day, orally, 3 times per week.

2. Sulfadiazine: 100 mg/kg per day (maximum 4g/day), orally, divided twice a day.

3. Folinic acid (leucovorin): 10 mg, orally, 3 times per week.

Note that due to theoretical risk of hyperbilirubinemia and kernicterus in newborns, some clinicians are concerned and do not recommend sulfadiazine use near delivery. Neonatologists should be informed that if maternaltherapy with sulfadiazine is maintained until near delivery, and a reduced dose three times weekly is preferred [19].

The recommendations for maternal treatment of toxoplasmosis in pregnancy is given in Table **1**.

Table 1. Summary of recommendations for maternal treatment of toxoplasmosis in pregnancy.

Maternal Toxoplasmosis Treatment		
Women with under 18 weeks of gestation at diagnosis.	Spiramycin is initiated and continued until PCR testing of amniotic fluid and obstetric ultrasound.	If PCR and ultrasound screening are negative, spiramycin should be taken until the end of gestation. If PCR is positive or fetal ultrasound is suggestive of congenital toxoplasmosis, the treatment should be switched to pyrimethamine-sulfadiazine plus folinic acid.
Women with more than 18 weeks of gestation at diagnosis.	Pyrimethamine-sulfadiazine plus folinic acid is initiated and continued until PCR testing of amniotic fluid and obstetric ultrasound.	If PCR and obstetric ultrasound screening are negative, spiramycin should be taken until the end of gestation. If PCR becomes positive or obstetric ultrasound becomes suggestive of congenital toxoplasmosis, the treatment should be maintained with pyrimethamine-sulfadiazine plus folinic acid.

OTHER POTENTIAL TREATMENT OPTIONS

There are limited studies in which a few drugs are being tested without proven safety and efficacy, these include the treatment of acute toxoplasmosis, for example: atovaquone (a cytochrome b inhibitor that inhibits oxidative phosphorylation and the respiratory chain), and sulfamethoxazole or sulfadiazine (which inhibit the biosynthesis of dihydropteroic acid [involved in folic acid synthesis] and act synergistically with trimethoprim, which inhibits the formation of tetrahydrofolic acid, essential for thymidine formation). Unfortunately, these drugs fail to eradicate the encysted and bradyzoites forms and are not recommended for treating pregnant women especially in the first trimester of gestation [10].

CONCLUSION

In conclusion, there is an urgent need to have safer drugs on hand that are a suitable for chemotherapy or prophylaxis in children and pregnant women, not only to eliminate the cystic stage of the parasite, but also to prevent relapses of toxoplasmosis.

Even in the absence of randomized placebo-controlled trials and with the urgent need of development of further researches on chemoprophylaxis to prevent congenital toxoplasmosis, we agree that there is enough evidence that supports the treatment of acute toxoplasmosis during pregnancy.

CONSENT FOR PUBLICATION

Not applicable.

CONFLICT OF INTEREST

The authors declare no conflict of interest, financial or otherwise.

ACKNOWLEDGEMENTS

Declared none.

REFERENCES

[1]   Bennett JE, Dolin R, Blaser MJ. Mandell, douglas, and bennett's principles and practice of infectious diseases. 8th ed., Philadelphia, PA: Elsevier/Saunders 2015.

[2]   Cortina-Borja M, Tan HK, Wallon M, *et al.* European multicentre study on congenital toxoplasmosis (EMSCOT). Prenatal treatment for serious neurological sequelae of congenital toxoplasmosis: an observational prospective cohort study. PLoS Med 2010; 7(10): e1000351.
[http://dx.doi.org/10.1371/journal.pmed.1000351] [PMID: 20967235]

[3]   Raeber PA, Biedermann K, Just M, Zuber P. Prevention of congenital toxoplasmosis in Europe. Schweiz Med Wochenschr Suppl 1995; 65: 96S-102S.
[PMID: 7716459]

[4]   Diesel AA, Zachia SA, Müller ALL, Perez AV, Uberti FAF, Magalhães JAA. Follow-up of toxoplasmosis during pregnancy: ten-year experience in a university hospital in southern brazil. Rev Bras Ginecol Obstet 2019; 41(9): 539-47.
[http://dx.doi.org/10.1055/s-0039-1697034] [PMID: 31546277]

[5]   Gontijo da Silva M, Clare Vinaud M, de Castro AM. Prevalence of toxoplasmosis in pregnant women and vertical transmission of toxoplasma gondii in patients from basic units of health from gurupi, tocantins, brazil, from 2012 to 2014. PLoS One 2015; 10(11): e0141700.
[http://dx.doi.org/10.1371/journal.pone.0141700] [PMID: 26558622]

[6]   Gras L, Gilbert RE, Wallon M, Peyron F, Cortina-Borja M. Duration of the IgM response in women acquiring Toxoplasma gondii during pregnancy: implications for clinical practice and cross-sectional incidence studies. Epidemiol Infect 2004; 132(3): 541-8.
[http://dx.doi.org/10.1017/S0950268803001948] [PMID: 15188723]

[7]   Brasil M da S. Insituto Sírio Libanês de Ensino e Pesquisa Protocolo de atenção Basica: Saúde das Mulheres. Brasília, DF: Ministério da Saúde 2016; p. 230.

[8]   Villard O, Breit L, Cimon B, et al. French national reference center for toxoplasmosis network. Comparison of four commercially available avidity tests for Toxoplasma gondii-specific IgG antibodies. Clin Vaccine Immunol 2013; 20(2): 197-204.
[http://dx.doi.org/10.1128/CVI.00356-12] [PMID: 23239801]

[9]   Ministério da Saúde Brasil. Protocolo de notificação e investigação: Toxoplasmose gestacional e congênita 2018. http://bvsms.saude.gov.br/bvs/publicacoes/protocolo_notificacao_%0Atoxoplasmose_gestacional.pdf

[10]   Rodriguez JB, Szajnman SH. New antibacterials for the treatment of toxoplasmosis; a patent review. Expert Opin Ther Pat 2012; 22(3): 311-33.
[http://dx.doi.org/10.1517/13543776.2012.668886] [PMID: 22404108]

[11]   Gilbert R, Gras L. European multicentre study on congenital toxoplasmosis. effect of timing and type of treatment on the risk of mother to child transmission of toxoplasma gondii. Int J Obstet Gynaecol 2003; 110(2): 20-112.
[http://dx.doi.org/10.1016/s1470-0328(02)02325-x]

[12]   Montoya JG. Systematic screening and treatment of toxoplasmosis during pregnancy: is the glass half full or half empty? Am J Obstet Gynecol 2018; 219(4): 315-9.
[http://dx.doi.org/10.1016/j.ajog.2018.08.001] [PMID: 30269768]

[13]   SYROCOT. Effectiveness of prenatal treatment for congenital toxoplasmosis: a meta-analysis of individual patients' data The. 2007; 369: 22-115.
[http://dx.doi.org/10.1016/S0140-6736(07)60072-5]

[14]   Prusa AR, Kasper DC, Pollak A, Gleiss A, Waldhoer T, Hayde M. The Austrian toxoplasmosis register, 1992-2008. Clin Infect Dis 2015; 60(2): e4-e10.
[http://dx.doi.org/10.1093/cid/ciu724] [PMID: 25216688]

[15]   Mandelbrot L, Kieffer F, Sitta R, et al. Prenatal therapy with pyrimethamine sulfadiazine vs spiramycin to reduce placental transmission of toxoplasmosis: a multicenter, randomized trial. Am J Obstet Gynecol 2018; 219(4): 7-9. 386

[16]   Montoya JG, Remington JS. Management of Toxoplasma gondii infection during pregnancy. Clin Infect Dis 2008; 47(4): 554-66.
[http://dx.doi.org/10.1086/590149] [PMID: 18624630]

[17]   Chaudhry SA, Gad N, Koren G. Toxoplasmosis and pregnancy. Can Fam Physician/ Le Médecin Fam Can 2014; 60: 6-334.

[18] Maldonado YA, Read JS. Diagnosis. Treatment, and Prevention of Congenital Toxoplasmosis in the United States. Pediatrics 2017; 139(2): e20163860.

[19] Kaplan JE, Benson C, Holmes KK, et al. Guidelines for prevention and treatment of opportunistic infections in HIV-infected adults and adolescents: recommendations from CDC, the National Institutes of Health, and the HIV Medicine Association of the Infectious Diseases Society of America. MMWR Recomm Rep 2009; 58(RR-4): 1-207; quiz CE1-4.

CHAPTER 9

Natural Anti-Infective Remedies In Pregnancy

Silvana Maria Zucolotto[*]

Medicine School, Federal Univ of Rio Grande do Norte, Natal, Brazil

Abstract: Natural remedies are widely used by pregnant women as they are perceived to be more "natural" and safe and also to avoid pharmaceutical treatment. Although some natural remedies can be used during pregnancy, some plants are not safe and for most of them, there is a lack of clinical evidence of safety. In addition, some natural remedies have a potential risk of herb-drug interactions. Many studies can be found in the literature, specifically on treating infections, but most are non-clinical studies. The main natural anti-infective remedies used by pregnant women are cranberry, *echinacea*, barberry, hydrastis, raspberry and garlic. The strongest clinical evidence was found in cranberry and *echinacea*, mainly to treat urinary tract infection recurrence and cold infection, respectively, these seem to be safe, but the efficacy is not clear. Natural remedies lack studies with methodological rigor conducted with standardized extracts with defined active compounds content for the guarantee of reliable results.

Keywords: Barberry, Cranberry, *Echinacea*, Efficacy, Garlic, Herbal Medicine, Hydrastis, Infection, Natural Product, Pregnancy, Red Raspberry, Safety.

BACKGROUND

Natural products have always performed an important role in drug discovery and natural remedies adopted as herbal medicines are widely used due to the belief that they are considered safe. The value of naturally derived drugs has increased considerably because of their efficacy and safety when compared to synthetic compounds [1, 2]. Some compounds originating from natural products (plants, marine organisms and microorganisms) are used until today, for example, morphine obtained from the latex of *Papaver somniferum* [3]. Another important finding was the discovery of the quinine alkaloid from the bark of *Cinchona*, which has been the only effective antimalarial treatment for almost 300 years [4]. Among natural remedies, medicinal plants are the most used, these include home preparations (for example: teas and decoctions) and herbal medicines [5].

---

[*] **Corresponding author Silvana Maria Zucolotto:** Medicine School, Federal Univ of Rio Grande do Norte, Natal, Brazil; Tel: +558433429818; E-mail: szucolotto@hotmail.com

Ricardo Ney Cobucci (Ed.)

The ancient use of medicinal plants is considered by laypersons as an indicator of safety [6]. In many cases drug interactions, reproductive toxicity and teratogenicity are not associated with their use, because the population believes that "natural remedies are entirely free of risks" [5]. However, it is important to clarify that they have a complex chemical composition, with some compounds being responsible for the pharmacological effect and others that may or may not be toxic. The lack of evidence of toxicity for some natural remedies cannot be considered an absence of toxicity [7, 8].

Herbal Medicines, unlike popular preparations, must guarantee constancy of quality, safe and efficacy. These products can have efficacy, safety and proven quality with well-defined indication and contraindication and known adverse effects, as much as traditional drugs, but this does not mean that they can be freely used by pregnant and lactating women [9].

However, when it comes to supplements or nutraceuticals you have to be careful with natural remedies, since even though they are marketed, it is not a drug and cannot be used to treat ailments. They may cause toxicity, have teratogenic and adverse effects, as well as be adulterated with non-official plant species or contain a mixture of a synthetic compound that is not associated with the extract [10].

In this sense, in the case of pregnant women, the use of natural remedies should be done very cautiously, using the following information.

Pregnancy and Natural Remedies

Pregnant women often use natural remedies due to the perception that they are natural and safer compared to traditional drugs [5, 8, 11, 12]. Natural remedies are used during pregnancy mainly to treat nausea and vomiting, reduce the risk of preeclampsia, shorten labour and treat common cold and urinary tract infection [13].

However, evidence is lacking about the potential harm of natural remedies used in pregnancy. Some scientific studies published in the literature have already shown the toxic potential of some natural remedies, such as teratogenicity, inducing contractions, increased risk of maternal bleeding and causing changes in neonatal hormones, due to the presence of compounds similar to hormones in natural remedies [5, 14]. Added to the lack of sufficient knowledge about the chemical compositions present in natural remedies and their efficacy and safety, the prescription of herbal medicines and even teas during pregnancy should be done with great caution and very carefully.

Pregnant women should inform the health professionals before consuming any natural remedies [13]. Great care should be taken with pregnant patients, mainly in the first three months in which the embryo is developing, and abnormalities can be induced by teratogenic agents, chemical, physical or biological. However, for each specific situation, the risks and benefits must be evaluated, even in the case of natural remedies. Generally, if the use of the natural remedies by pregnant women has demonstrated negative effects on the women or fetus, its use is contraindicated. In the case of natural remedies that have few or no clinical evidences it is suggested that it should be used with caution under the supervision of a health care practitioner [5, 14].

Natural Anti-infective Remedies in Pregnancy

Anti-infective remedies are among the most common drugs used during the pregnancy. As seen in previous chapters of this book, the choice of an anti-infective drug during pregnancy should ensure safe use for both mother and fetus, even if it is a natural remedy that lacks clinical studies. In addition to the possible adverse effects, as is the case for synthetic drugs, for natural remedies, pharmacokinetic changes of the gestational period should be considered [15, 16]. Specifically with herbs, there are a lack of pharmacokinetic knowledge, since the extracts are complex chemical mixtures and not an isolated compound, as is the case with traditional drugs.

The potential risks and benefits of natural remedies for pregnant women and the fetus are difficult to assess and few clinical trials have been found in the literature [11, 14].

The following brief reviews that are presented are on certain herbals remedies that have presented reports as natural anti-infective remedies used by pregnant women. Species included in the review are cranberrry, *echinacea*, barberry, hydrastis, raspberry, and garlic. In view of this, the purpose of this chapter is to gather the available information on benefits and untoward effects of natural remedies used during pregnancy.

Cranberry (Vaccinium macrocarpon, Vaccinium oxycoccos)

The species *Vaccinium macrocarpon* Aiton belongs to the family Ericaceae. It has the synonym of the scientific name *V. oxycocos* and is widely distributed throughout Europe and United States. It is popularly known as cranberry [17].

It is very common during pregnancy for a woman to have asymptomatic urinary tract infection (UTI), which may cause some problems for the mother and fetus [18], these problems include premature labor, rupture of membranes, spontaneous abortion, chorioamnionitis, postpartum endometritis, post-menstrual wound infections, post-surgical infections, and subclinical pelvic inflammatory disease [16]. One of the alternative treatments quoted in the literature to treat UTI in pregnant women is the use of cranberry juice and/or capsules and cranberry extract tablets.

Some nonclinical studies have shown that the proanthocyanidins and fructose compounds described in cranberry act on bacterial adherence to the urinary tract epithelial cells [19 - 23], but do not seem to interfere in bacteria already adhered to those cells [24].

In a systematic review published in 2012, different cranberry products (in juice or as capsules/tablets) compared to placebo groups showed no benefit in most intervention groups, and the observed benefits were very small. Many withdrawals from some of the studies (mainly in groups that consumed juice) suggests that cranberry products may not be acceptable over long periods of time. When tablets and capsules were tested, few of the studies reported the content of the marker (active principle or analytic chemical compound) of the tablets or capsules that were used. A criticism is that the cranberry can only be recommended when standardized extract is used with the content of the marker. This systematic review identified 24 studies (total of 4473 participants) comparing cranberry products with control or alternative treatments. The review reported that the use of cranberry products in tablets and capsules may be indicated only for women with recurrent UTIs, and only if they contain the recommended amount of proanthocyanidins (at least 36 mg/d). The results demonstrate that the use of cranberries for preventing urinary tract infections may decrease the number of symptomatic UTIs over a 12-month period [25].

Specifically in regard to pregnant women, in this systematic review only two studies were included (659 participants) [26, 27]. The first study was a study comparing a single daily dose (240 mL) or two (480 mL) or three (720 mL) daily doses of cranberry juice with a placebo beverage [26]. In another clinical trial a higher daily dose (1000 mL) was evaluated of cranberry juice with the same volume of water in placebo group [27]. The current body of evidence for studies in pregnant women suggest that cranberry juice is not effective in reducing UTIs in pregnant women. It is important to mention that both clinical trials with pregnant women were performed with cranberry juice and not capsules/tablets. Also, both had a high number of withdrawals (39% and 28%, respectively).

Regarding safety evaluation of cranberry products, a cohort study was conducted in Norway with mothers and children born between 1999 and 2008 and a systematic review was published subsequently that has already been mentioned. Pregnant women between weeks 17 and 30, and 6 months after the birth were questioned and information about pregnancy outcomes was retrieved from the Norwegian Medical Birth Registry. As a result it was observed that of 68,522 women included in the study, 919 (1.3%) used cranberry during pregnancy, it was not possible to observe any increased risk of congenital malformations related to the use of cranberry. In addition, the use of cranberry was also not associated with the following risks to pregnant women and the baby: increased neonatal fetal death, low birth weight, small baby stature for gestational age, prematurity, low Apgar score (<7), and maternal vaginal bleeding in first trimester of pregnancy [28].

Another recent study also evaluated the safety and tolerability of daily use of cranberry by pregnant women with asymptomatic bacteriuria. Women with less than 16 gestational weeks were randomized into two groups, one group received two cranberry capsules (n=24), dose equivalent to 250 mL of cranberry juice, or placebo capsules (content capsule: at least 16.25 mg of proanthocyanidins) (n=25), twice daily. Eleven participants were excluded from the study and from the total of 38 patients, the results were similar between those who received cranberry capsules and placebo. The majority of pregnant women stopped using cranberry after 34–38 weeks. 30% of patients withdrew for different reasons, but only 1 withdrew due to intolerance to the cranberry capsules. Seven cases of asymptomatic bacteriuria occurred in 5 patients: 2 out of 24 (8%) in the cranberry group and 3 out of 25 (12%) in the placebo group. No cases of cystitis or pyelonephritis were observed [29].

Previous studies suggest a possible interaction between cranberry and the anticoagulant warfarin [30, 31].

It is unknown whether ingestion of cranberry may increase the risk of bleeding in vulnerable patient groups, *e.g.* pregnant women. In addition, a report suggests that cranberry interacts with diazepam and diclofenac by pharmacokinetics *via* inhibition of cytochrome P450 enzymes (inhibition of CYP2C9). This herb-drug interaction can increase levels of drugs metabolized by this enzyme [32].

Based on the current literature, although the safety of cranberry use during pregnancy needs further investigations, its was defined as "safe for use" in pregnancy [13]. Taken together, clinical evidences with women patients suggest that cranberry can be helpful in decreasing UTI recurrence, but the evidence to support its effectiveness in UTI treatment in pregnancy is still weak. Moreover, as

UTIs may have negative effects on pregnancy, it is important that antibiotics are used to treat UTIs and that natural remedies are not used as an alternative to treatment, but as a complement [8]. The recommended dose based in studies is from 250 to 1000 mL/day of juice or capsules containing extracts (at least 18mg of proanthocyanidins) twice a day.

Echinacea

This species is widely used in some European countries and in North America for common colds. *Echinacea* preparations available on the market contain different species and parts of the plant, different extraction methods (dried raw material, alcoholic extract or juice from fresh plants) and sometimes mixture with other plants [33]. The more common *Echinacea* species used are *E. angustifolia*, *E. purpurea* and *E. pallida*. The more common names are American cone flower, black Sampson and black Susan [34].

The major secondary metabolites described in *Echinacea* are caffeic acid derivatives, such as echinocoside, cichoric acid, cynarin, polysaccharides, glycoproteins and alkamides [35].

A systematic review evaluated 24 randomized controlled clinical trials with 4631 participants that used different *Echinacea* preparations in intervention groups for preventing and treating common colds or induced rhinovirus infections compared to placebo. Due to differences in the *Echinacea* preparations evaluated, it was difficult reach strong conclusions. Only five trials were rated as having a low risk of bias. The risk of bias of the trials was rated from low to high. The majority of clinical trials investigated whether the use of *Echinacea* preparations after the onset of cold symptoms shortens the duration of illness, compared with placebo. Some preparations seem be more effective than a placebo for treating colds, but the overall evidence for treatment effects is still weak (6 clinical trials reported data about the duration of colds, but only 3 showed benefits in groups that were treated with *Echinacea* compared with placebo). According to clinical trials investigating *Echinacea* in the prevention of colds no reductions in illness occurrence were shown. However, almost all prevention clinical trials indicated small preventive effects. The number of withdrawals or adverse effects did not differ significantly between control and treatment groups, in both prevention and treatment trials, but in prevention trials more withdrawals were observed due to untoward events in the treatment groups [33].

A Canadian study investigated the safety of use of *Echinacea* by pregnant women. A *Teratogenic Information Service* contacted four hundred and twelve pregnant women between 1996 and 1998 and asked them about use of *Echinacea* during the pregnancy. Two hundred and six of them had taken *Echinacea* during pregnancy, while the other 206 (the control group) subsequently decided not to take it. In the *Echinacea* group, 112 women (54%) reported taking the plant in the first trimester of pregnancy and 17 (8%) used it during pregnancy. No significant differences were observed between groups in relation to congenital defects, nor were there differences in the outcome of pregnancy, delivery method, maternal weight gain, gestational age, fetal weight or fetal distress [36].

Regarding the safety of *Echinacea* in pregnancy, more recently a study evaluated the possible consequences of the use of *Echinacea* on malformations of the baby and untoward effects during gestation. The Norwegian Mother and Child Cohort Study (MoBa) was used, which counted on a total of 68,522 women and their children. Data was obtained from three self-administered questionnaires answered by pregnant women between 17- 30 weeks and 6 months after birth. Of the total number of women, 363 (0.5%) responded that they had used *Echinacea* during pregnancy. These women were characterized by advanced age and delivery before 2002 and, for a lower percentage, smoking during pregnancy [37]. The use of *Echinacea* has not been associated with an increased risk of malformation. The recommended dose is 5-10 mL of *Echinacea* tincture [13].

Barberry (Berbery vulgaris)

The *Berbery vulgaris* species belongs to the Berberidaceae family and is widely distributed in Europe and Asia. It is commonly known as barberry [17].

Regarding the chemical composition of *B. vulgaris*, the presence of isoquinolinic alkaloids such as berberine, oxyananthine, berbamine, palmatine, jatorrizine, columbamine and tannins have been described [38].

The products used with *B. vulgaris* are usually commercialized as berberine-rich extract from *B. vulgaris*. In the literature some scientific evidence was found of the use of *B. vulgaris* in treatment of upper respiratory tract infection [34], however, these were non clinical studies and were conducted with the alkaloid berberine isolated and not with de *B. vulgaris* extract, as can be observed in the review [39]. This discrepancy makes it difficult to evaluate the results. In addition to this, a systematic review was not found, only a few clinical trials. It is important to mention that no studies were found on the use of berberine and *B. vulgaris* extract in pregnant women.

There is also evidence of the use of *Berbery vulgaris* to treat resistant chloroquine cases of malaria, however, there was only one clinical trial. A clinical trial evaluated the combination of pyrimethamine in combination with berberine, tetracycline or cotrimaxazol in clearing the parasite. A clinical trial randomized two hundred and fifteen patients with chloroquine-resistant malaria into three groups. The first group (82 patients) received pyrimethamine and berberine (berberine group), the second group (64 patients) were treated with pyrimethamine and tetracycline (tetracycline group) and the third group (69 patients) received pyrimethamine and cotrimoxazole (cotrimoxazole group). The berberine group showed the best response for chloroquine resistant malaria patients [40].

In addition, a randomized clinical trial of 80 married women (18–40 years old) with bacterial vaginosis evaluated the efficacy of vaginal gel of *B.vulgaris* (5%; in metronidazole base) (n=40) compared with only metronidazole vaginal gel (0.75%) (n=40). *B. vulgaris* group had a better response than the metronidazole gel alone (p<0.001). The patients treated with *B. vulgaris* with a metronidazole gel base did not show relapse, but in the metronidazole group, 30% of patients had relapse during three weeks' follow-up. Therefore, the association of *B. vulgaris* with metronidazole was more effective in the treatment of bacterial vaginosis [41].

However, because it is a complex mixture of secondary metabolites, possible adverse effects have been described (based on an *in vivo* study) related to the use of *B. vulgaris* by pregnant women due to the presence of the alkaloid berberine. According to the results of a non-clinical study in rats, berberine can cause neonatal jaundice (kernicterus). In this study, berberine displaced bilirubin bound to albumin when administered at a dose of 10-20 IU /g *via* i.p. daily for 1 week. After this time, a decrease in serum bilirubin protein binding was observed. Persistent elevation in serum concentrations of total and unbound bilirubin was also observed [42]. Other evidence, based on scientific technical literature, reports that berberine may cause uterine stimulation [34, 43]. No recommended daily dose was found.

Hydrastis canadenses

Hydrastis canadenses belongs to the Ranunclaseae family. It is commonly known as goldenseal [17].

H. canadensis, as with *B. vulgaris*, has in its chemical composition the presence of isoquinolinic alkaloids such as hydrastine, berberine, tetrahydroberberastine, berberastine, canadaline canalidine, canadine, hydrastinine and β-hydrastine [44, 45].

For the *H. canadensis* species, there are also clinical evidences to treat chloroquine cases resistant to malaria [40] and infectious diarrhea [46]. However, it is important to comment that these clinical studies [40, 46] were conducted with the alkaloid berberine and not with *H. canadenes* extract. Therefore it is not possible to extrapolate on the efficacy observed for the isolated compound to the extract.

Considering the presence of the alkaloid berberine in *H. canadenses* extract, the same possible adverse effects described for *B. vulgaris* are valid for *H.canadensis*. No recommended daily dose was found.

Red Raspberry (Rubus idaeus)

Rubus idaeus (Rosaceae) is commonly known as red raspberry. Its leaves are used as uterine tonic to promote labour with little bleeding and as an astringent to treat diarrhoea. The raspberry leaves had higher contents of catechin, epigallocatechin gallate, rutin, ferulic acid, chlorogenic acid and *p*-hydroxybenzoic acid compared to blackberry leaf samples [47].

According to two clinical trials, a positive association was observed with red raspberry use in treating diarrhoea. The effect can be related to tannins present in this species. The daily recommended dose is 1.5–5 g [13]. Red raspberry use appears to be a low risk for pregnant women and the baby.

In a randomized clinical trial, 192 women (32 weeks of gestation) received 1.2 g of raspberry leaf tablets twice daily. In the outcome of the study no untoward effects to mothers or babies were reported, a shortening in the second stage of labour and a lowering of the rate of forceps delivery was also observed. A retrospective observational study conducted on 108 pregnant women showed that 57 women who used raspberry leaves showed less frequency of an artificial rupture of membranes or the need to have caesarean section, forceps or vacuum birth compared to 51 controls [48, 49].

Garlic (Allium sativum L.)

Allium sativum is commonly known as garlic, a perennial herb cultivated in different countries. It is commonly used as a food ingredient, spice and the extract of plant is used as herbal medicine [17]. Allicin is an organosulfur compound mainly found in garlic after mastication or crushing of the raw material [49].

In vivo and *in vitro* studies of antimicrobial and antifungal effects showed that allicin interacts with thiol groups and this justifies, at least in part, their properties [50]. There is a lack of clinical evidence, but its use seems safe in woman pregnant [51].

Other important evidence is that supplementation with garlic during pregnancy can reduce the risk of preeclampsia and protein retention in urine. A randomized clinical trial evaluated garlic tablet supplementation (800 mg/day) or placebo on preeclampsia with 100 primigravida during the third trimester of pregnancy. The untoward effects reported were the garlic odor and in some patients, nausea. The study did not identify any incidence of malformations in newborn infants and there were no spontaneous abortions [51]. However, excessive use of garlic should be avoided in early pregnancy, in pregnant women with thyroid disorders and before surgery, including caesarean, because it may interfere with blood clotting. Another adverse effect of using garlic during pregnancy is that it may increase heartburn.

CONCLUSION

The scarcity of clinical trials to evaluate the efficacy and safety of natural anti-infective remedies in pregnancy and the poor quality of some clinical trials may explain why the conclusions are generally elusive or contradictory. For the medicinal plants in the studies, there is a lack of some important information, such as the scientific name of the plants, part of the plant, extraction method (solvent, ratio of plant), content of the marker in each product (juice, capsules or tablets), and daily dose. In addition it is not possible to extrapolate on the results obtained with an isolated compound to a rich-extract. Extracts are complex mixtures of chemical compounds. The potential benefits of the natural anti-infective remedies for pregnant women are difficult to assess and very few clinical trials have been published in the literature. On the other hand, the use of the plants reviewed here appears to be safe in pregnant women. Cranberry can be helpful for reducing UTI recurrence in women; however, the evidence to support its effectiveness in UTI treatment during pregnancy is weak, but safe. The use of *Echinacea* to treat the common cold indicates that it is safe and can offer a small improvement that needs to be better investigated. In the use of hydrastis and barberry to treat resistant chloroquine cases of malaria there is a lack of clinical trials. Raspberry can be used as an astringent in the case of diarrhoea and its use seems safe. Garlic/allicin have antimicrobial effect observed in *in vitro* and *in vivo* studies and its use during the pregnancy is considered safe. Lastly, it is important to develop clinical trial studies with capsules containing standardized extract with defined active compound content to identify adverse events during pregnancy and the postnatal period.

CONSENT FOR PUBLICATION

Not applicable.

CONFLICT OF INTEREST

The authors declare no conflict of interest, financial or otherwise.

ACKNOWLEDGEMENTS

Declared none.

REFERENCES

[1]   Shams Ul Hassan S, Jin HZ, Abu-Izneid T, Rauf A, Ishaq M, Suleria HAR. Stress-driven discovery in the natural products: A gateway towards new drugs. Biomed Pharmacother 2019; 109: 459-67. [https://doi.org/10.1016/j.biopha.2018.10.173]. [http://dx.doi.org/10.1016/j.biopha.2018.10.173] [PMID: 30399582]

[2]   Newman DJ, Cragg GM. Natural products as sources of new drugs over the nearly four decades. J Nat Prod 2020; 83(3): 770-803. [http://dx.doi.org/10.1021/acs.jnatprod.9b01285]

[3]   Viegas C Jr, Bolzani V, Barreiro EJ. The natural products and the modern medicinal chemistry. Quim Nova 2006; 29(2): 326-37. [http://dx.doi.org/10.1590/S0100-40422006000200025].

[4]   Ganesan A. The impact of natural products upon modern drug discovery. Curr Opin Chem Biol 2008; 12(3): 306-17. [https://doi.org/10.1016/j.cbpa.2008.03.016]. [http://dx.doi.org/10.1016/j.cbpa.2008.03.016] [PMID: 18423384]

[5]   Bruno LO, Simoes RS, de Jesus Simoes M, Girão MJBC, Grundmann O. Pregnancy and herbal medicines: An unnecessary risk for women's health-A narrative review. Phytother Res 2018; 32(5): 796-810. [https://doi.org/10.1002/ptr.6020]. [http://dx.doi.org/10.1002/ptr.6020] [PMID: 29417644]

[6]   Frawley J, Adams J, Steel A, Broom A, Gallois C, Sibbritt D. Women's use and self-prescription of herbal medicine during pregnancy: an examination of 1,835 pregnant women. Womens Health Issues 2015; 25(4): 396-402. [https://doi.org/10.1016/j.whi.2015.03.001]. [http://dx.doi.org/10.1016/j.whi.2015.03.001] [PMID: 25935822]

[7]   Fong HH. Integration of herbal medicine into modern medical practices: issues and prospects. Integr Cancer Ther 2002; 1(3): 287-93. [https://doi.org/10.1177/153473540200100313]. [http://dx.doi.org/10.1177/153473540200100313] [PMID: 14667286]

[8]   Kennedy DA, Lupattelli A, Koren G, Nordeng H. Safety classification of herbal medicines used in pregnancy in a multinational study. BMC Complement Altern Med 2016; 16: 102. [https://dx.doi.org/10.1186/s12906-016-1079-z]. [http://dx.doi.org/10.1186/s12906-016-1079-z] [PMID: 26980526]

[9]   Carvalho ACB, Lana TN, Perfeito JPS, Silveira D. The Brazilian market of herbal medicinal products and the impacts of the new legislation on traditional medicines. J Ethnopharmacol 2018; 212: 29-35. [https://doi.org/10.1016/j.jep.2017.09.040]. [http://dx.doi.org/10.1016/j.jep.2017.09.040] [PMID: 28987598]

[10]   Moreira DL, Teieira SS, Monteiro MHD, de-Oliveira AC A X, Paumgartten FJR. Traditional use and safety of herbal medicines. Rev Bras Farmacogn 2014; 24(2): 258-7. [http://dx.doi.org/10.1016/j.bjp.2014.03.006]

[11]   Ernst E. Herbal medicinal products during pregnancy: are they safe? BJOG 2002; 109(3): 227-35. [http://dx.doi.org/10.1111/j.1471-0528.2002.t01-1-01009.x] [PMID: 11950176]

[12]   Westfall RE. Herbal medicine in pregnancy and childbirth. Adv Ther 2001; 18(1): 47-55. [http://dx.doi.org/10.1007/BF02850250] [PMID: 11512532]

[13]   Laelago T. Herbal medicine use during pregnancy: Benefits and untoward effects. IntecOpen 2018; pp. 103-19. [http://dx.doi.org/10.5772/intechopen.76896]

[14]   Louik C, Gardiner P, Kelley K, Mitchell AA. Use of herbal treatments in pregnancy. Am J Obstet Gynecol 2010; 202(5): 439.e1-439.e10.
[http://dx.doi.org/10.1016/j.ajog.2010.01.055] [PMID: 20452484]

[15]   Gwee A, Cranswick N. Anti-infective use in children and pregnancy: current deficiencies and future challenges. Br J Clin Pharmacol 2015; 79(2): 216-21.
[http://dx.doi.org/10.1111/bcp.12363] [PMID: 24588467]

[16]   Yudin MH. Bacterial vaginosis in pregnancy: diagnosis, screening, and management. Clin Perinatol 2005; 32(3): 617-27.
[http://dx.doi.org/10.1016/j.clp.2005.05.007] [PMID: 16085023]

[17]   Tropicos. 2019. https://www.tropicos.org/

[18]   Schneeberger C, Geerlings SE, Middleton P, Crowther CA. Interventions for preventing recurrent urinary tract infection during pregnancy. Cochrane Database Syst Rev 2012; 11: CD009279.
[http://dx.doi.org/10.1002/14651858.CD009279.pub2] [PMID: 23152271]

[19]   Sobota AE. Inhibition of bacterial adherence by cranberry juice: potential use for the treatment of urinary tract infections. J Urol 1984; 131(5): 1013-6.
[http://dx.doi.org/10.1016/S0022-5347(17)50751-X] [PMID: 6368872]

[20]   Habash MB, Van der Mei HC, Busscher HJ, Reid G. The effect of water, ascorbic acid, and cranberry derived supplementation on human urine and uropathogen adhesion to silicone rubber. Can J Microbiol 1999; 45(8): 691-4.
[http://dx.doi.org/10.1139/w99-065] [PMID: 10528401]

[21]   Zafriri D, Ofek I, Adar R, Pocino M, Sharon N. Inhibitory activity of cranberry juice on adherence of type 1 and type P fimbriated *Escherichia coli* to eucaryotic cells. Antimicrob Agents Chemother 1989; 33(1): 92-8.
[http://dx.doi.org/10.1128/AAC.33.1.92] [PMID: 2653218]

[22]   Howell AB, Botto H, Combescure C, *et al.* Dosage effect on uropathogenic *Escherichia coli* anti-adhesion activity in urine following consumption of cranberry powder standardized for proanthocyanidin content: a multicentric randomized double blind study. BMC Infect Dis 2010; 10: 94.
[http://dx.doi.org/10.1186/1471-2334-10-94] [PMID: 20398248]

[23]   Foo LY, Lu Y, Howell AB, Vorsa N. A-Type proanthocyanidin trimers from cranberry that inhibit adherence of uropathogenic P-fimbriated *Escherichia coli*. J Nat Prod 2000; 63(9): 1225-8.
[http://dx.doi.org/10.1021/np000128u] [PMID: 11000024]

[24]   Lowe FC, Fagelman E. Cranberry juice and urinary tract infections: what is the evidence? Urology 2001; 57(3): 407-13.
[http://dx.doi.org/10.1016/S0090-4295(00)01100-6] [PMID: 11248607]

[25]   Jepson RG, Williams G, Craig JC. Cranberries for preventing urinary tract infections. Cochrane Database Syst Rev 2012; 10(10): CD001321.
[http://dx.doi.org/10.1002/14651858.CD001321.pub5]

[26]   Essadi F, Elemehashi MO. Efficacy of cranberry juice for the prevention of urinary tract infections in pregnancy [abstract]. Poster Session. J Matern Fetal Neonatal Med 2010; 23(1): 378.
[https://doi.org/10.3109/14767051003802503].

[27]   Wing DA, Rumney PJ, Preslicka CW, Chung JH. Daily cranberry juice for the prevention of asymptomatic bacteriuria in pregnancy: a randomized, controlled pilot study. J Urol 2008; 180(4): 1367-72.
[http://dx.doi.org/10.1016/j.juro.2008.06.016] [PMID: 18707726]

[28]   Heitmann K, Nordeng H, Holst L. Pregnancy outcome after use of cranberry in pregnancy--the Norwegian Mother and Child Cohort Study. BMC Complement Altern Med 2013; 13: 345.
[http://dx.doi.org/10.1186/1472-6882-13-345] [PMID: 24314317]

[29]   Wing DA, Rumney PJ, Hindra S, Guzman L, Le J, Nageotte M. Hindra s, Guzman L, Le J, Nageotte M. Pilot study to evaluate compliance and tolerability of cranberry capsules in pregnancy for the prevention of asymptomatic bacteriuria. J Altern Complement Med 2015; 21(11): 700-6.
[http://dx.doi.org/10.1089/acm.2014.0272] [PMID: 26535612]

[30]   Hamann GL, Campbell JD, George CM. Warfarin-cranberry juice interaction. Ann Pharmacother 2011; 45(3): e17.
[http://dx.doi.org/10.1345/aph.1P451] [PMID: 21364039]

[31]   Mohammed Abdul MI, Jiang X, Williams KM, *et al.* Pharmacodynamic interaction of warfarin with cranberry but not with garlic in healthy subjects. Br J Pharmacol 2008; 154(8): 1691-700.
[http://dx.doi.org/10.1038/bjp.2008.210] [PMID: 18516070]

[32]   McLay JS, Izzati N, Pallivalapila AR, *et al.* Pregnancy, prescription medicines and the potential risk of herb-drug interactions: a cross-sectional survey. BMC Complement Altern Med 2017; 17(1): 543.
[http://dx.doi.org/10.1186/s12906-017-2052-1] [PMID: 29258478]

[33]   Karsch-Völk M, Barrett B, Kiefer D, Bauer R, Ardjomand-Woelkart K, Linde K. *Echinacea* for preventing and treating the common cold. Cochrane Database Syst Rev 2014; 2: CD000530.
2014.https://www.ncbi.nlm.nih.gov/pubmed/24554461
[http://dx.doi.org/10.1002/14651858.CD000530.pub3]

[34]   Mills E, Dugoua JJ, Perri D, Koren G. Herbal medicines in pregnancy and lactation: An evidence-based approach. Boca Raton: Taylor and Francis Medical 2006; p. 368.
[http://dx.doi.org/10.1201/b13984]

[35]   Manayi A, Vazirian M, Saeidnia S. *Echinacea purpurea*: Pharmacology, phytochemistry and analysis methods. Pharmacogn Rev 2015; 9(17): 63-72.
[http://dx.doi.org/10.4103/0973-7847.156353] [PMID: 26009695]

[36]   Gallo M, Sarkar M, Au W, *et al.* Pregnancy outcome following gestational exposure to *echinacea*: a prospective controlled study. Arch Intern Med 2000; 160(20): 3141-3.
[http://dx.doi.org/10.1001/archinte.160.20.3141] [PMID: 11074744]

[37]   Heitmann K, Havnen GC, Holst L, Nordeng H. Pregnancy outcomes after prenatal exposure to *echinacea*: the Norwegian Mother and Child Cohort Study. Eur J Clin Pharmacol 2016; 72(5): 623-30.
[http://dx.doi.org/10.1007/s00228-016-2021-5] [PMID: 26895223]

[38]   Mokhber-Dezfuli N, Saeidnia S, Gohari AR, Kurepaz-Mahmoodabadi M. Phytochemistry and pharmacology of berberis species. Pharmacogn Rev 2014; 8(15): 8-15.
[http://dx.doi.org/10.4103/0973-7847.125517] [PMID: 24600191]

[39]   Imenshahidi M, Hosseinzadeh H. Berberine and barberry (*Berberis vulgaris*): A clinical review. Phytother Res 2019; 33(3): 504-23.
[http://dx.doi.org/10.1002/ptr.6252] [PMID: 30637820]

[40]   Sheng WD, Jiddawi MS, Hong XQ, Abdulla SM. Treatment of chloroquine-resistant malaria using pyrimethamine in combination with berberine, tetracycline or cotrimoxazole. East Afr Med J 1997; 74(5): 283-4.
[PMID: 9337003]

[41]   Masoudi M, Kopaei MR, Miraj S. Comparison between the efficacy of metronidazole vaginal gel and *Berberis vulgaris* (*Berberis vulgaris*) combined with metronidazole gel alone in the treatment of bacterial vaginosis. Electron Physician 2016; 8(8): 2818-27.
[http://dx.doi.org/10.19082/2818] [PMID: 27757195]

[42]   Chan E. Displacement of bilirubin from albumin by berberine. Biol Neonate 1993; 63(4): 201-8.
[http://dx.doi.org/10.1159/000243932] [PMID: 8513024]

[43] Farnsworth NR, Bingel AS, Cordell GA, Crane FA, Fong HH. Potential value of plants as sources of new antifertility agents I. J Pharm Sci 1975; 64(4): 535-98.
[http://dx.doi.org/10.1002/jps.2600640404] [PMID: 167146]

[44] Mahady GB, Pendland SL, Stoia A, Chadwick LR. *In vitro* susceptibility of *Helicobacter pylori* to isoquinoline alkaloids from *Sanguinaria canadensis* and *Hydrastis canadensis*. Phytother Res 2003; 17(3): 217-21.
[http://dx.doi.org/10.1002/ptr.1108] [PMID: 12672149]

[45] Weber HA, Zart MK, Hodges AE, *et al*. Method validation for determination of alkaloid content in goldenseal root powder. J AOAC Int 2003; 86(3): 476-83.
[http://dx.doi.org/10.1093/jaoac/86.3.476] [PMID: 12852562]

[46] Rabbani GH, Butler T, Knight J, Sanyal SC, Alam K. Randomized controlled trial of berberine sulfate therapy for diarrhea due to enterotoxigenic *Escherichia coli* and *Vibrio cholerae*. J Infect Dis 1987; 155(5): 979-84.
[http://dx.doi.org/10.1093/infdis/155.5.979] [PMID: 3549923]

[47] Pavlovic AV, Papetti A, Zagorac DCD, *et al*. Phenolics composition of leaf extracts of raspberry and blackberry cultivars grown in Serbia. Ind Crops Prod 2016; 87: 304-14.
[http://dx.doi.org/10.1016/j.indcrop.2016.04.052]

[48] Simpson M, Parsons M, Greenwood J, Wade K. Raspberry leaf in pregnancy: Its safety and efficacy in labor. J Midwifery Womens Health 2001; 46(2): 51-9.

[49] Parsons M, Simpson M, Ponton T. Raspberry leaf and its effect on labour: safety and efficacy. Aust Coll Midwives Inc J 1999; 12(3): 20-5.
[http://dx.doi.org/10.1016/S1031-170X(99)80008-7] [PMID: 10754818]

[49] Salehi B, Zucca P, Orhan IE, *et al*. Allicin and health: A comprehensive review. Trends Food Sci Technol 2019; 86: 502-16.
[http://dx.doi.org/10.1016/j.tifs.2019.03.003]

[50] Groppo F, Ramacciato J, Motta R, Ferraresi P, Sartoratto A. Antimicrobial and antifungal activity of garlic. Int J Dent Hyg 2007; 5(2): 109-15.
[http://dx.doi.org/10.1111/j.1601-5037.2007.00230.x] [PMID: 17461963]

[51] Ziaei S, Hantoshzadeh S, Rezasoltani P, Lamyian M. The effect of garlic tablet on plasma lipids and platelet aggregation in nulliparous pregnants at high risk of preeclampsia. Eur J Obstet Gynecol Reprod Biol 2001; 99(2): 201-6.
[http://dx.doi.org/10.1016/S0301-2115(01)00384-0] [PMID: 11788172]

SUBJECT INDEX

dermatitis 94
diarrhea 158
   syndromes 22
Infectious diseases 17, 74, 110, 132, 134
   congenital 17
   specialists and obstetricians 110
Influenza 64, 97
   infection 64
   syndrome 97
Influenza virus 9, 10
   maternal 10
Inhibition 28, 48, 54, 66, 90, 121, 155
   enzymatic 121
   metabolic induction/enzymatic 28
   protease dimerization 121
Inhibitors 39, 50, 63, 79, 95, 124, 125, 148
   beta-lactamase 79
   dehydropeptidase 50
   integrase strand transfer 124
   integrin 63
   non-nucleoside reverse transcriptase 63
   nucleoside reverse transcriptase 39
   nucleotides reverse transcriptase 39
   topoisomerase 95
Intolerance 50, 79, 155
   alcohol 50
Intravaginal clindamycin cream 57

K

Kidneys 24, 26, 27, 28, 36, 50, 51, 53, 77
   fetal 28
   ultrasonography 77

L

Lactic 114, 133
   acid 133
   acidosis 114
Lactobacillus 133, 135
   crispatus 133
   iners 133
   jensenii 133
   johnsonii 133
Lipodystrophy 122
Listeria 50, 58
   monocytogenes 58
Liver 49, 58
   abscess 49

disease 58

M

Macrolides 29, 30, 32, 33, 35, 45, 54, 55, 81
   semisynthetic 33
Malaria 11, 64, 157, 158, 160
   chloroquine-resistant 158
   severe falciparum 65
Malaria infection 65
Malformations 4, 33, 62, 97, 118, 124, 146,
     155, 157, 160
   cardiac 4
   congenital 33, 155
   neural tube 124
Mammary glands 26
Maternal 3, 7, 8, 9, 32, 39, 136
   diagnosis 7, 8
   immunity 2, 136
   immunodeficiency 39
   infection, symptomatic 9
   rubella infection 3
   serum cephalosporin levels 32
Meningitis 7, 14, 15, 31, 49, 52, 101
   aseptic 14
   bacterial 49
   syphilitic 101
Meningoencephalitis 8
Metamorphosis 120
Methemoglobinemia 47
Methicillin-resistant *Staphylococcus aureus*
     (MRSA) 51, 52, 58
Metropolitan atlanta congenital defects
     program (MACDP) 116, 120
Michigan Medicaid program 37
Middle 9, 33
   cerebral artery (MCA) 9
   ear infections 33
Miscarriage 15, 22, 25, 57, 62, 65, 89, 91,
     119, 120, 136, 137
   late 136
   rate 91, 120
   risk of 22, 62
Modifications 27, 80, 95, 102, 134
   biochemical 26
   physiological 102
Most HPV infections 89
Mutations 56, 114, 117, 119, 121, 122, 125,
     126
   resistant 117

T

U

V

www.ingramcontent.com/pod-product-compliance
Lightning Source LLC
Chambersburg PA
CBHW041704210326
41598CB00007B/529